M000271876

Lower Body Training

The Definitive Guide to Increasing Size, Strength, and Athletic Performance

Jason Brown, MS, CSCS

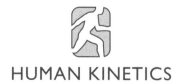

HUMAN KINETICS

Library of Congress Cataloging-in-Publication Data

Names: Brown, Jason, 1983- author.
Title: Lower body training : the definitive guide to increasing size,
  strength, and athletic performance / Jason Brown, MS, CSCS.
Description: Champaign, IL : Human Kinetics, [2023] | Includes
  bibliographical references.
Identifiers: LCCN 2021038099 (print) | LCCN 2021038100 (ebook) | ISBN
  9781718206878 (Paperback) | ISBN 9781718206885 (ePub) | ISBN
  9781718206892 (PDF)
Subjects: LCSH: Physical education and training. | Physical
  fitness--Physiological aspects. | Exercise.
Classification: LCC GV711.5 .B77 2023 (print) | LCC GV711.5 (ebook) | DDC
  796.071--dc23/eng/20211202
LC record available at https://lccn.loc.gov/2021038099
LC ebook record available at https://lccn.loc.gov/2021038100

ISBN: 978-1-7182-0687-8 (print)

Copyright © 2023 by Jason Brown

Human Kinetics supports copyright. Copyright fuels scientific and artistic endeavor, encourages authors to create new works, and promotes free speech. Thank you for buying an authorized edition of this work and for complying with copyright laws by not reproducing, scanning, or distributing any part of it in any form without written permission from the publisher. You are supporting authors and allowing Human Kinetics to continue to publish works that increase the knowledge, enhance the performance, and improve the lives of people all over the world.

To report suspected copyright infringement of content published by Human Kinetics, contact us at **permissions@hkusa.com**. To request permission to legally reuse content published by Human Kinetics, please refer to the information at **https://US.HumanKinetics.com/pages/permissions-information**.

This publication is written and published to provide accurate and authoritative information relevant to the subject matter presented. It is published and sold with the understanding that the author and publisher are not engaged in rendering legal, medical, or other professional services by reason of their authorship or publication of this work. If medical or other expert assistance is required, the services of a competent professional person should be sought.

The web addresses cited in this text were current as of September 2021, unless otherwise noted.

Acquisitions Editors: Michael Mejia and Michelle Earle; **Developmental Editor:** Laura Pulliam; **Managing Editor:** Hannah Werner; **Copyeditor:** Christina T. Nichols; **Permissions Manager**: Dalene Reeder; **Graphic Designer:** Denise Lowry; **Cover Designer:** Keri Evans; **Cover Design Specialist:** Susan Rothermel Allen; **Photograph (cover):** Peter Muller/Image Source/Getty Images; **Photographs (interior)**: © Human Kinetics; Photos on pages 51, 52, 91, 106, 107, 108, 119, 129, 130, 198, 200, 201, 202, 212, 213, 214, 215, 216, 217, 226, 227, 228, 229, 230, 231, 239, 243, and 249 © Jason Brown; **Photo Production Specialist**: Amy M. Rose; **Photo Production Manager:** Jason Allen; **Senior Art Manager**: Kelly Hendren; **Illustrations:** © Human Kinetics, unless otherwise noted; **Printer:** Versa Press

We thank Crunch Fitness in Champaign, Illinois, for assistance in providing the location for the photo shoot for this book.

Printed in the United States of America   10 9 8 7 6 5 4 3 2 1

The paper in this book is certified under a sustainable forestry program.

Human Kinetics
1607 N. Market Street
Champaign, IL 61820
USA

United States and International
Website: **US.HumanKinetics.com**
Email: info@hkusa.com
Phone: 1-800-747-4457

Canada
Website: **Canada.HumanKinetics.com**
Email: info@hkcanada.com

E8335

Tell us what you think!
Human Kinetics would love to hear what we can do to improve the customer experience. Use this QR code to take our brief survey.

I'd like to dedicate this book to my wife, Dani Brown,
who has been a constant beacon of positivity
and support in the quest to reach my goals
as a coach, husband, and father.

CONTENTS

EXERCISE FINDER

Chapter 6 Hip-Dominant Exercises (continued)

Chapter 7

(continued)

FOREWORD

Movement, exercise, strength, and conditioning—they are a science and an art. To master them, one needs both theoretical and experiential knowledge. I first met Jason in 2016 while teaching a workshop about movement assessment at the gym he owned at the time. Since then, I've had the pleasure of working with him both personally and professionally, having interviewed him for *The Movement Fix* podcast several times, developed a training program together, and gotten suggestions for my own body and my own training.

I've had the opportunity to ask him pointed questions, watch firsthand how he writes training programs, and witness his authenticity behind closed doors. There is no fluff with Jason—he practices what he preaches. He goes the extra mile, is detail oriented, and is always looking for ways to improve his methods and techniques. Typically, theoretical and practical knowledge come in separate packages. It's rare for someone to have the depth of theoretical knowledge Jason has about strength training while simultaneously having real-world, practical experience. And his practical experience comes not only from training others and writing programs for gyms but from applying his knowledge personally to his own body. There is no truer test than successfully implementing what you teach. It's pure authenticity.

Since I was 12 years old, I've been strength training in one way or another. Over the 22 years since, I've been learning and refining applications in my own life and the lives of others. Training, getting stronger, and managing the complexities of the human body are not always straightforward, and there is ample misinformation available that can lead you down the wrong path. I am thrilled to see Jason authoring *Lower Body Training*. The world needs more resources like this one, which compiles conceptual understanding and real-world experience into a book that you can read and apply to yourself and to those you train.

This book will provide you with understanding that you might not have gotten otherwise. Going through this book, studying the materials, and applying them will change the way you approach lower body strength training—for the better. This is a resource you will refer back to over and over, seeing new layers of wisdom and experience each time you go through it.

Thank you, Jason, for putting in the time and energy to not only find what really works but also gather that knowledge together so others can apply and benefit from it. I am honored to call you a friend and a colleague and could not be more impressed with your accomplishments thus far. I look forward to seeing the impact this book has on both the professionals who read it and those who reap the benefits in their training and experience positive changes in their lives.

—*Ryan DeBell, MS, DC*

ACKNOWLEDGMENTS

I would like to thank Chad Waterbury for recommending me for this book as well as the support and advice he has provided throughout my career. I would also like to thank Louie Simmons for being an innovator and challenging me to be a better coach! Finally, I would like to thank Christopher Swart, PhD, for assisting with the anatomy section of this book as well as helping me to continue my own education in the field of exercise science.

INTRODUCTION

Over the past decade, coaches have shifted lower body training away from basic foundational patterns such as squatting, lunging, and hip hinging, putting new twists on these classics by using different equipment such as landmines and kettlebells and by introducing accommodating resistance (AR) to elicit different training effects. Tools like AR have the ability to alter the strength curve of these variations to change the relative load through a full range of motion (ROM). Though these approaches are novel, they still reinforce the basic foundational patterns of squatting, lunging, and hip hinging while allowing variability in exercise selection as proficiency increases. As more variations are added to the list of lower body exercises, if you are more advanced in your training, you can expect to see new gains in movement proficiency, add lean muscle mass, and improve strength qualities.

However, adding exercise variation requires a complex knowledge of the lower body—each exercise must have a purpose for its inclusion other than novelty. It's important to have at least a basic understanding of the different types of strength training. For example, in order to choose exercises that align with the intent of a given training session, you should fully understand how qualities such as maximal strength differ from qualities such as speed strength. At the base of all true strength training, maximal strength connects to nearly every other biomotor ability, including strength endurance, speed strength, strength speed, and explosive strength.

This book will introduce you to lower body exercise variations that will give you the ability and knowledge to develop strength on a number of levels. Exercise variability will always be a key component for avoiding the biological law of accommodation (also called detraining), but there should be a line between too much exercise variability and not enough; we will cover this more thoroughly in part III of this book when we dive into the programs. Exercise variability and avoidance of accommodation, the two key principles of effective program design, are closely related and should be properly managed so that you are still able to improve motor patterns in keystone foundational patterns (squat, lunge, and hip hinge) while incurring positive training adaptations for both movement patterns and performance (through metrics such as maximal strength).

You may tend to go down the exercise selection rabbit hole, constantly varying your exercises and always looking for the next best exercise, but this book will help you dial in your selection of lower body exercise variations with choices that will elicit positive adaptations while avoiding creating compensation patterns. Instilling improper motor patterns is a hallmark of overdoing exercise variation without first building the proper foundational patterns. Of course, experimentation is part of the individual training process—because no two exercises are created the same way and no two exercises will resonate the same with each individual—but being able to consolidate that list of variations will eliminate a fair amount of guesswork. In turn, this will empower you to choose exercises that are easy to implement, keep your training interesting by challenging your muscles in novel ways, and do not exacerbate common imbalances.

Throughout the book, we will focus on developing the lower body and the keystone foundational movements of the squat, lunge, and hip hinge. However, we will not underplay the importance of individual muscle development through targeted isolation exercise because this allows you to isolate individual imbalances and lagging muscle groups. When it comes to improving multijoint patterns in terms of strength development, single-joint exercises are an incredibly effective means for improving muscular deficits.

You will also be introduced to different types of strength modalities that will have a profound effect on your ability to develop strengths from a general, specific, and maximal strength standpoint. This will lead to gains in absolute strength, which is your ability to generate maximal force and torque regardless of bodyweight. We will also introduce the basic principles of functional anatomy for the foundational patterns, which will allow you to better understand proper programming in terms of volume, sequence, and frequency.

The squat, lunge, and hip hinge patterns have always been an instrumental aspect of my clients' training plans. I've also come to the conclusion that although no two individuals present the same on paper in terms of limitations and movement proficiency, these foundational movements are a mainstay for just about anyone regardless of their goals and background. What's even more interesting is that the patterns that tend to cause localized pain and exacerbate nagging pains in people I've worked with (for most, the hip hinge pattern) are typically the same movements that have the most significant effect on health and wellness. Lower body issues are all too common as lower back disorder statistics continue to rise at alarming rates. Movements like the Romanian deadlift (RDL) variations play a key role in learning (or relearning) how to properly perform the hip hinge pattern, building strength in key areas to help mitigate lower body issues. Performance gains are also routine when squats, lunges, and hip hinges are mainstays in program design. As the old adage goes, *You cannot build a house without a proper foundation.*

Once you have mastered these patterns with bodyweight only, it's logical to add resistance in the form of dumbbells, kettlebells, barbells, or a landmine; these exercise progressions are provided in parts II and III of this book. Many of my clients have incurred significant benefits from improving the ratio of strength between their posterior (glute complex, upper body complex, and hamstrings) and anterior (quadriceps) musculature. Direct posterior chain training has always been an integral part of effective program design for improving strength, performance, and aesthetics. In this book, you will find no shortage of great exercise variations that will enable the development of key musculature to support effective movement in both everyday living and the field of play. The training programs in this book spend a fair amount of time developing the musculature of the hamstrings, glutes, and spinal erectors, but you should still expect to see exercises dedicated to improving anterior musculature such as the quadriceps.

This book should leave you with a firm grasp of both how to *program* effective lower body training exercises and how to properly *sequence* (order of movements in a training day) these movements into a training plan. You will learn to distribute volume correctly among different exercise variations and to understand the *why* behind each specific exercise selection in your own training plan. Understanding the deeper meaning of any movement in a training plan affords this movement the right to be in your plan in the first place—make no mistake, random exercise selection leads to haphazard results and overuse injury. Strength and conditioning professionals operating without a well-thought-out plan should be avoided at all costs.

TAKING BACK THE DREADED LEG DAY

For years, leg day at commercial gyms has been viewed negatively and lower limb exercises are often neglected altogether or poor selections are used for lower limb exercises. Instead, training "plans" usually contain high doses of machines. While machines can certainly bring an advantage in conjunction with squat and hinge variations, if the use of machines is the only exposure one has to lower limb development, then improvements in cross-sectional muscle mass and thereby in maximal strength will be limited.

Why is training of the legs dreaded by so many, particularly men? The obvious answer for many is that it subjects them to their own insecurities about lack of leg strength. This shortcoming can be tough on one's ego, but the only way to get better is to stop avoiding squats and deadlifts. I'll give people the benefit of the doubt and list a lack of knowledge of how to effectively program big movement patterns as another big reason people avoid lower body training. In addition, a lack of movement proficiency leads people to believe that if they train these patterns heavily they'll likely get injured. And last but not least, these patterns induce a fair amount of pain when trained with a full ROM. Multijoint movements are globally demanding patterns, using high-energy fuel sources such as phosphocreatine, and their effects on the muscular system and the cardiorespiratory system are obvious and felt by anyone attempting them. With that said, recovery between sets should be longer (anywhere between two and four minutes) in order to replace high-energy phosphates and have the ability to reproduce similar levels of output, but this isn't common knowledge for the average gym-goer, who doesn't have a baseline understanding of bioenergetics.

While casual exercisers certainly find machines more accessible, they would likely have more success if they first learned the core lifts. (Hiring a qualified coach would be a great place to start.) This would then allow them to focus more on movements like the front squat and RDL variations as the mainstay in their training, followed by supplemental work, which could include the use of machines to support their goals while improving potential imbalances. A great training plan will use healthy doses of assistance exercises such as single-joint movements to improve muscular asymmetries, induce muscular hypertrophy, and balance the demand on the nervous system. (Multijoint movements are much more demanding on the central nervous system [CNS] than single-joint exercises.) Conversely, multijoint patterns like the front squat and RDL are important, but even these variations have their effective doses, and simply doing more will not lead to better results.

Prioritizing only multijoint movements such as squats and hip hinges can be counterproductive if volume and frequency are not managed as well—too much of a good thing can certainly have the reverse effect and lead to overtraining or an overuse injury, and because multijoint movements are more demanding on the body, there is more chance of breakdown. For example, if your only lower limb training comes by way of the front squat and RDL, both patterns are bilateral, meaning we are asking both legs to work in conjunction with one another, while other muscles are working isometrically to stabilize when these patterns are being performed. While bilateral work is a huge part of the training equation, unilateral work is equally important. Unilateral exercises such as the lunge, single-leg RDL, and split squat variations will be keystone assistance exercises to help improve muscular imbalance, induce muscular hypertrophy, and give you the power to perform higher volumes of work in a given session with less overall cost on the CNS. This will allow you to train optimally and improve your weakest muscle groups with less chance of overtraining.

Lower limb training is arguably the single most important aspect of a training plan because it sets the stage (and foundation) for all other aspects of training to be built on. One key tenet to understand in developing lower limb training plans is that while the foundational patterns of squatting, lunging, and hinging are intrinsically great patterns, the *dose* and *frequency* should be properly managed: More is not better; better is better. As previously mentioned, it's important to understand how to supplement your training with smaller, single-joint exercises or functional resistance machines that, when used appropriately, will have a profound effect on hypertrophic adaptations (muscle growth) as well as strength endurance qualities. Another key tenet is allowing for proper recovery between sessions. It is vital to understand the cost of multijoint movements in terms of fatigue on the CNS. Overall, when lower body training is effectively managed, you can expect to see gains in strength from a variety of standpoints (maximal strength and strength endurance) and even in hormone production.

PART I

THE SCIENTIFIC APPROACH TO LOWER BODY TRAINING

Chapter 1

Meet the Muscles

A basic understanding of how the musculature of the lower body works and functions is paramount to effectively programming lower limb exercises in a diverse and balanced way. A deeper understanding of the basic anatomy will allow you to better analyze limitations and imbalances, will help you avoid overuse injuries, and can help you design programs that will expedite recovery after higher-threshold training sessions.

This chapter will cover the basics of primary and secondary movers—the musculature that is responsible for driving human movement. Though this text will not delve as deeply as an anatomy text, I want to provide the "basics" so you are able to identify limitations while also understanding better how to strategically target different muscle groups. For instance, it's not uncommon for hip shifts to present when maximal loads are used with a movement such as a squat variation. Hip shifts are quite common with bilateral movements such as the squat and occur when the hips shift laterally during the concentric phase of the squat pattern. Although it's nearly impossible to eliminate all muscular imbalances, you can assume that with bilateral training these imbalances will only be exacerbated. Instead, we look to unilateral exercises to provide the basis for improving current limitations. As a result, the level of hip shift that may present with maximal loads in the squat can be decreased, but more importantly, the level of strength in agonist and antagonist muscle groups can be improved, which directly correlates to improving muscle size.

QUADRICEPS

Since the quadriceps are located at the front of the body, this compels many people to dedicate a fair amount of time to their development, just as people often prioritize their chest training over their upper

3

back. While there are benefits to having strong and massive quadriceps, from a health and longevity standpoint, development of the posterior musculature presents many benefits over spending your time focusing solely on the quadriceps. (We'll spend a fair amount of time developing the reasoning behind this later in chapter 6 when hip-dominant exercises are discussed.) However, understanding the anatomical makeup of the quadriceps is important so you can accurately assess which aspects of your quadriceps will need the most attention; this will allow you to make better decisions with regard to exercise selection.

The quadriceps femoris, located in the anterior (extensor) compartment of the thigh, is made up of four parts—rectus femoris, vastus lateralis, vastus medialis, and vastus intermedius (see figure 1.1). The quadriceps muscle covers the majority of the anterior surface and the sides of the thigh. The rectus femoris, the only part of the quadriceps that crosses the hip joint and therefore plays a role in both knee and hip flexion, is located in the middle of the anterior compartment of the thigh. The rectus femoris is superficial, covering the vastus intermedius. In addition, the rectus femoris also covers the superior-medial portion of both the vastus lateralis and vastus medialis. In Latin, the word *rectus* means "straight," and the rectus femoris is named for its anatomical position: running straight down the center of the anterior compartment of the thigh. It originates from the anterior inferior iliac spine and from the superior edge of the acetabulum.

The three vastus portions of the quadriceps lie deep under the rectus femoris, originate from the body of the femur, and span the trochanters to the condyles. The vastus lateralis, located on the lateral (outer) portion of the thigh, away from the midline of the body, originates from the greater trochanter and linea aspera of the femur. The vastus medialis, located on the medial (inner) portion of the thigh, closest to the midline of the body, originates from the linea aspera of the femur. Lastly, the vastus intermedius is located deep to the rectus femoris muscle, between the vastus medialis and vastus lateralis, and originates from the anterior and lateral surfaces of the femur. The four parts of the quadriceps merge together at their

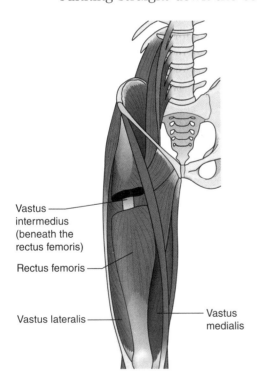

Vastus intermedius (beneath the rectus femoris)

Rectus femoris

Vastus lateralis

Vastus medialis

Figure 1.1   The quadriceps muscles.

distal ends to form the quadriceps tendon at the patella and attach to the tibial tuberosity via the patellar ligament.

All four quadriceps muscle parts are innervated by the femoral nerve and are responsible for extending the leg at the knee joint. Only the rectus femoris plays an additional role in flexing the thigh at the hip joint. The collective action of the quadriceps muscle parts makes them all important knee extensors and therefore paramount in daily activities such as walking, running, jumping, cycling, and even squatting and lunging. The additional role of the rectus femoris—assisting the iliopsoas in hip flexion—is important not only for performance but also for everyday activities. The rectus femoris is active during two distinct phases of the gait (walking) cycle. In the first phase the rectus femoris is important during the loading phase when all four muscle parts act eccentrically at the knee during load-bearing activities such as walking or running. During the swing phase of the walking or running cycle, the rectus femoris plays a key role, acting as a hip flexor to propel the trailing leg forward into the swing phase for the following step. During activities such as walking, all four quadriceps parts (as well as ligaments and tendons) are responsible for stabilizing the patella and keeping it in place. If the patella moves out of place during activities such as walking, it is commonly referred to as *patella tracking disorder*. This can occur by either lateral or medial displacement of the patella.

When we're considering direct training of the quadriceps, it is important to know that the quads will respond well to many rep ranges and frequencies of training because their muscle fiber makeup is mixed. Certain areas of the quadriceps, such as the vastus intermedius, are composed of more fast-twitch muscle fiber. This makes the case that in order to effectively train the quadriceps, one should use rep ranges that satisfy multiple special strengths, such as submaximal strength ranges of three- to six-rep max, traditional hypertrophy ranges of 6- to 12-rep max, and a strength endurance range of 15 or more repetitions. Common staple exercises to train the quadriceps are lunge and split squat variations, as well as bigger bilateral movements like the front squat or Anderson squat variations, which will be highlighted in chapter 5.

Understanding the function and anatomy of the quadriceps is a great place to start for program design and for those who may be lacking strength or symmetry (or both) in the quadriceps. This will allow you to make progressive improvements to your quadriceps in a 12- to 16-week time frame. Furthermore, having a grasp on optimal programming specific to quadriceps is important not only for aesthetics but for everyday function because quadriceps strength can be directly linked to knee health. (Knee injury is common with endurance activities such as jogging that many use as their primary means of training.)

HAMSTRINGS

The three muscles of the posterior (flexor) compartment of the thigh, known as the hamstrings, are the semitendinosus, semimembranosus, and biceps femoris (see figure 1.2). The hamstrings get their name because their elongated tendons are stringlike. The three hamstring muscles play an important role in the actions of hip extension and knee flexion. The biceps femoris is a unique muscle of the hamstring group because it has two heads (long and short). The long and short head of the biceps femoris have different sites of origin but do have the same insertion point. The long head of the biceps femoris is more superficial compared to the short head; if you looked at the muscles from a posterior view, the short head would be mostly blocked from view. The short head of the biceps femoris originates at the linea aspera of the femur (lower down the leg than other hamstring muscles). For this reason, it is sometimes not included as part of the hamstring group since originating at the ischial tuberosity is considered a defining characteristic of the hamstring group. Furthermore, due to its site of origin, the short head of the biceps femoris only crosses the knee joint and therefore plays a role only in knee flexion and not in hip extension. It is important to note that the short head of the biceps femoris can be completely absent in some individuals.

The hamstrings flex the knee joint and extend the thigh to the back side of the body. They are used in walking, sprinting, and many other movements. All the hamstring muscles, with the exception of the short head of the biceps femoris, have their origin (where their tendons attach to bone) at the ischial tuberosity of the hip. As previously mentioned, the short head of the biceps femoris actually originates further down the leg, on the linea aspera of the femur. The most medial muscle, the semimembranosus, inserts on the medial condyle of the tibia bone. The semitendinosus inserts on the superior part of the medial tibia. The most lateral hamstring, the biceps femoris, inserts on the lateral side of the fibula and attaches to the superior part of the lateral tibia. An important anatomical landmark is located in the posterior portion of the knee and is called the popliteal fossa. This landmark is a diamond-shaped space formed by the tendons of the biceps femoris muscle, which create the lateral border, and the tendons of

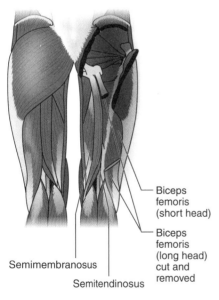

Biceps femoris (short head)

Biceps femoris (long head) cut and removed

Semimembranosus

Semitendinosus

Figure 1.2 The hamstring muscles.

the semimembranosus and semitendinosus, which create the medial border. Lastly, the semitendinosus, semimembranosus, and the long head of the biceps femoris are all innervated by the tibial branch of the sciatic nerve, whereas the short head of the biceps femoris is innervated by the common fibular branch of the sciatic nerve.

The hamstrings play a crucial role in many daily activities such as walking, running, and jumping and in controlling some movement in the glutes. The muscles that make up the hamstrings are known as *biarticular muscles* because they cross and influence movement at two joints: the hip and the knee joints. Biarticular muscles are typically found in the upper and lower extremities. Let's briefly look at the actions of each hamstring muscle. First, the long head and short head of the biceps femoris have similar but slightly different actions. The long head is responsible for flexion of the knee, extension of the hip, and lateral rotation of the lower leg, and it can also assist in lateral rotation of the thigh when the hip is extended. On the other hand, the short head of the biceps femoris (which has a different origin than all the other hamstring muscles) is responsible for flexion of the knee as well as lateral rotation of the lower leg when the knee is slightly flexed. The main actions of the semitendinosus muscle (which receives its name due to having a long tendon of insertion) are knee flexion, hip extension, and medial rotation of the lower leg when the knee is flexed. The semitendinosus also plays a small role in medial rotation of the thigh at the hip joint. Another important anatomical landmark worth mentioning is the pes anserinus, which means "goose foot" in Latin—it's a name that reflects its resemblance to the foot of a goose. The pes anserinus, a common area of pain and inflammation, is formed by the attachment of three muscles in the same location (semitendinosus, sartorius, and gracilis) proximally on the medial side of the tibia and superficial to the medial collateral ligament (MCL) of the knee. Lastly, the primary actions of the semimembranosus are knee flexion, hip extension, and medial rotation of the thigh and lower leg.

The hamstrings play an important role during the different phases of walking or running. As mentioned previously, the hamstrings are primarily involved in hip extension and knee flexion. During walking or running, the hamstrings also play a key role in eccentrically slowing down both hip flexion and knee extension before the heel strikes the ground.

The hamstrings are composed of a high degree of fast-twitch muscle fiber, which will vary based on the genetic makeup of the individual. To develop the fast-twitch muscle fiber of the hamstrings, I recommend training with heavier loads in the three- to six-rep max range. The hamstrings also respond favorably to true maximal strength work with singular effort one-rep maxes. Training the hamstrings in submaximal strength settings is not common, though, and many stick to standard hypertrophy schemes in the 8- to 15-rep range, which is a mistake. Common exercise variations to optimally train the hamstrings are RDL variations, rack pull deadlift variations, and glute-ham raise variations.

CALVES

The group of seven muscles in the posterior compartment of the lower leg is commonly referred to as the *calves*. This group can be further subdivided into three superficial muscles and four deep muscles. The gastrocnemius and soleus are the two most dominant muscles and make up the shape of the calves (see figure 1.3). Both are superficial muscles and are heavily involved in plantar flexion (pointing the foot downward). The gastrocnemius is the most superficial and is most prominent in forming the shape of the posterior compartment of the lower leg. The gastrocnemius has two heads that originate from the left and right femoral condyle, respectively, and merge together to form a single muscle belly that runs down the whole posterior of the lower leg. It combines with the soleus to form the calcaneal (Achilles) tendon, which inserts on the calcaneus (heel bone).

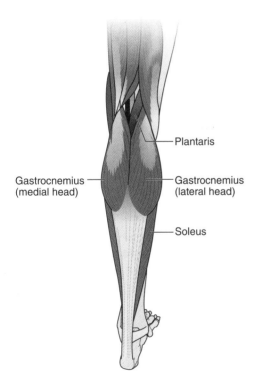

Gastrocnemius
(medial head)

Plantaris

Gastrocnemius
(lateral head)

Soleus

Figure 1.3 The calf muscles.

The broad and flat soleus muscle is located beneath the gastrocnemius and gets its name from its resemblance to a sole, which is a flat fish. The soleus originates at the head of the fibula and medial border of the tibia. Similar to the gastrocnemius, the soleus also inserts on the calcaneus via the calcaneal tendon. Both the gastrocnemius and the soleus are important in plantar flexion and are innervated by the tibial nerve. The gastrocnemius and soleus are commonly grouped together and referred to by anatomists as the *triceps surae*.

The calves can be isolated by performing movements involving plantar flexion (pointing the toes down). The two major categories of calf exercises are those that maintain an extended knee and those that maintain a flexed knee. The first category includes movements such as standing calf raises and the second category includes movements such as seated calf raises. Movements with a straight knee (such as the standing calf raise) will target the gastrocnemius muscle more, and movements with a bent knee (such as the seated calf raise) will target the soleus muscle more. However, both variations will target both muscles to a large degree.

It is worth mentioning that both the gastrocnemius and soleus play an important role in the skeletal-muscle pump. The term *skeletal-muscle pump* refers to certain muscles' ability to aid in the circulation of blood through the cardiovascular system. When someone is standing, gravity tends to pull blood to the periphery of the body (in this case, the lower leg). When someone is upright but moving, the gastrocnemius and soleus contract to help push blood back to the heart. The movement of blood back to the heart is called *venous return*. The calf muscles help push blood back to the heart and therefore aid in the heart's ability to effectively pump blood throughout the remainder of the body.

Because the calf muscles are composed predominantly of slow-twitch muscle fiber, they respond well to high-frequency training and higher-volume sets of 15 or more repetitions. The calves also use the stretch-shortening cycle. The stretch-shortening cycle is what allows for an increase in force and power production if a rapid eccentric countermovement is immediately followed by an explosive concentric movement. Think of a vertical jump in which there is a rapid eccentric countermovement; elastic energy is stored within the tendon and can be immediately released if a quick concentric muscle action follows, thus increasing force and power for a higher jump. In other words, the calves have the potential to use the energy created through the eccentric phase of the exercise variation (e.g., a calf raise) to their advantage. Because of this, to achieve full benefits when training the calves, it is best to pause between repetitions to allow the calves to bear the brunt of the work. Common calf exercises include seated calf raises, single-leg dumbbell calf raises, and standing calf raises with a barbell in the back rack position (placed on the mid traps as is done for a high-bar back squat).

GLUTE COMPLEX

The glute complex, located posteriorly to the pelvic girdle at the proximal end of the femur, is made up of three muscles—the gluteus maximus, the gluteus medius, and the gluteus minimus (see figure 1.4). The glute complex plays an important role in movements such as walking, running, jumping, and many other athletic tasks. Originating at the iliac crest, sacrum, and coccyx, the gluteus maximus spans the buttocks at about a 45-degree angle and inserts into the iliotibial tract and the gluteal tuberosity just below the greater trochanter of the femur. The gluteus

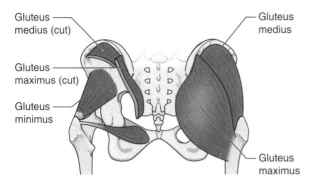

Gluteus medius (cut)

Gluteus maximus (cut)

Gluteus minimus

Gluteus medius

Gluteus maximus

Figure 1.4 The gluteal muscles.

maximus, the predominant muscle in forming the shape of the buttocks, is not only the largest of the three gluteal muscles but also one of the largest muscles in the body overall. As the most superficial of all three glute complex muscles, the gluteus maximus is the primary extensor of the hip, pulling the pelvis backward, in addition to its role in lateral rotation of the thigh. The quadrilateral-shaped gluteus maximus covers the other two muscles of the glute complex except for a small portion of the gluteus medius—a spot that is a common site for intramuscular injections. The gluteus medius is a fan-shaped muscle located between the gluteus maximus and gluteus minimus and is responsible for abduction and medial rotation of the leg. Both the gluteus medius and the gluteus minimus originate on the ilium of the hip bone and insert at the greater trochanter of the femur. Finally, the gluteus minimus is the smallest and deepest of the glute complex muscles and, like the gluteus medius, is responsible for abduction and medial rotation of the leg. The gluteus maximus is innervated by the inferior gluteal nerve, whereas both the gluteus medius and gluteus minimus are innervated by the superior gluteal nerve.

The functions of the glutes include extension and abduction, and they also perform internal and external rotation of the hip joint. The gluteus maximus supports the extended knee. The glutes respond to a high amount of slow-twitch fiber muscle like the calves, making the optimal schemes for training them in the higher ranges (10 or more repetitions). Staple exercises to train the glutes include the barbell glute bridge, barbell glute hip thrust, and 45-degree back raise.

Functional anatomy as it relates to lower body training is complex, to say the least, but this basic information will allow your programming for lower body–specific training days to be more targeted and thus optimized in terms of delivery, execution, and long-term effectiveness. While it may seem that pulling together a list of solid lower body exercises discussed in this book is simple enough, I'd urge you to first consider your individual goals, where you're most limited with regard to lower limb development, and how you can reach your goals while simultaneously achieving health and longevity.

Chapter 2

Create Better Balance Through Movement

It's no secret that we are living in a society plagued by chronic conditions such as lower back disorders, generalized front-sided shoulder pain, and obesity. For many, lower back pain occurs through no fault of their own. The daily postures of most—that is, sitting in flexion, internal rotation, and adduction—present many issues for people that only exacerbate their current issues. Lower back disorders are more connected to these daily postures than most would suspect. In fact, one study found that gluteus medius weakness and gluteal muscle tenderness are common symptoms in people with chronic nonspecific lower back pain (Cooper et al. 2016). Although this finding is not particularly surprising to most fitness professionals (I've seen it for the past decade), it gives these professionals the unique opportunity to profoundly affect their clients' health and wellness through strength training, particularly training that focuses on the proper use of quad- versus hip-dominant movements as well as hip adduction and abduction.

UNDERSTANDING THE BILATERAL VERSUS UNILATERAL TRAINING DEBATE

In strength and conditioning circles, it is common knowledge that one needs to have a balance between bilateral movements (e.g., multijoint movements like squats and deadlifts) and unilateral movements (e.g., single-joint movements like lunges). There is no debate there, but a commonly asked question is how much of each should make up one's training program. First, let's try to understand the consequences of taking on only one of these forms as stand-alone training, or engaging in a program that neglects unilateral movements and focuses more on their bilateral counterparts. This is a common theme in many training programs today such as CrossFit or Olympic weightlifting. If the programming of bilateral movements such as squats and deadlifts makes up the bulk of your training, there certainly could be positive adaptations made, but the question is, for how long would these positive adaptations occur? For most people in this situation, which is common in functional fitness communities, there will be setbacks due to phenomena such as bilateral asymmetries and bilateral deficits.

First off, a bilateral asymmetry is a discrepancy in strength between right and left limbs. Of course, no two limbs are created perfectly equal, so this makes sense, but too high of doses of bilateral movements will exacerbate these discrepancies instead of remedying them. A bilateral deficit occurs when there are asymmetries in force production between unilateral and bilateral movements (Haff 2016). An easy example of this would be performing a one-rep max of a split squat variation, taking the sum of both legs, and comparing that to a bilateral max, such as for a back squat. While this may not be a reliable test for everyone and involves high levels of motor control, the point is that trained athletes want to see some semblance of balance between the right and left limbs. However, please note that while many well-established coaches have used this test as a marker of lower body strength symmetry, the reliability of this test may not be consistent with real-world data. It is possible to have an athlete test poorly for unilateral strength yet exhibit high levels of bilateral strength.

At Westside Barbell (WSBB), considered the "strongest gym in the world," they follow the 80/20 rule—80 percent of their training volume is made up of "special exercises"—assistance exercises performed with dumbbells and unilateral movements—while the other 20 percent comes from the classic bilateral lifts and their variations (Simmons 2015). You may be thinking, "How is this the strongest gym in the world when it comes to the squat, bench press, and deadlift considering they *only* perform these variations 20 percent of the time?" The answer is resoundingly simple—"We use special exercises to build lean-muscle mass, improve imbalances and lagging muscle-groups, and improve upon our weakest links—we are only as strong as our weakest link" (Simmons 2015). Of course, the athletes who train at WSBB are always technicians when it comes to squatting, pressing, and pulling, so spending the bulk of their time building where they are weak makes sense, but assistance work is still vitally important for the average person while building component motor patterns with the squat and hinge patterns.

Furthermore, given the physiology of unilateral movements, it makes sense that we are able to better address limitations and imbalances with them since we are able to train our lower body in isolation with less contribution of opposing limbs (most times). Lastly, an important consideration is the central nervous system (CNS) fatigue that is created by performing multijoint movements. For instance, if I asked a client to squat and deadlift for their entire 60-minute training session, not only would this create tissue damage, but the CNS fatigue could take up to 96 hours to fully recover from. If you do not consider these aspects of training and only train with movements that result in high levels of CNS fatigue, your risk of overtraining will be higher. Conversely, if the dose of multijoint movements is commensurate with the dose of single-joint assistance exercises within the same session, the demand on the CNS will be reduced, thus allowing for better recovery between sessions of both the CNS and the peripheral nervous system.

It's commonplace to see higher-level athletes pushing their squat and pulling volume and neglecting the less "sexy" components of training such as single-joint exercises. This yields a greater chance of creating compensatory motor patterns that could result in an overuse injury and— because bilateral movements apply more stress to the CNS—higher levels of fatigue. The fatigue may manifest with lesser-known symptoms such as loss of motivation (French 2016). In other words, higher doses of bilateral movements present many challenges to the CNS and the musculoskeletal system. Practitioners who prescribe high doses of bilateral movements frequently are increasing the risk of overtraining among their clients, so a balance between bilateral and unilateral work must be achieved, with the latter being prescribed in higher doses than the former to prevent deleterious effects and to create symmetry in the lower body. This will also increase the chances of creating synergistic training effects by way of keeping stress in check.

In short, the balance between bilateral and unilateral movements is paramount to your success. It's important to understand that you can push the volume of unilateral exercises more than you can for bilateral exercises since the demand on the CNS and the likelihood of ingraining compensation patterns are lower. With that said, the increase in anabolic hormones from bilateral movements is greater than from single-joint exercises, so you would not want to completely disregard bilateral movements. The key takeaway is applying balance relative to the individual. As noted, WSBB athletes are masters of the squat and pull and need more specificity to bring up lagging muscle groups, whereas beginners may still need to devote time to simply developing the motor pattern of their squat and pull. Because the nuances of individual programming can differ so much from individual to individual, everyone requires an individualized approach to effective training long term.

ACHIEVING BALANCE THROUGH PROPER MOVEMENT PATTERNS

It makes sense to devote a significant amount of time to strength training the regions of the posterior chain such as the glutes, hamstrings, and spinal erectors when they are underdeveloped (or, for many, simply not functioning properly), even if you don't suffer from lower back pain. This effectively counters many of these issues by bringing people into more extension, external rotation, and abduction movements, and it provides a small countermeasure of relief from everyday postures many find themselves in for hours on end. (A staggering portion of the population spends the majority of their lives sitting in flexion-based postures.)

You will notice that this book spends a great deal of time systematically training the musculature of the posterior regions of the body. This is because daily postures of most people not only present structural problems but also create lack of strength in this key musculature, which allows compensation and faulty motor patterns to be ingrained and causes an overreliance on vulnerable areas of the body in everyday movement. For example, due to a lack of ability to load the hamstrings when picking up an object (as a result of weak hamstrings and poor motor control), that load is then relegated to the lumbar spine, or lower back, with little contribution from the glutes and hamstrings. Picking up an object without loading the hamstrings is akin to teaching a client to deadlift without learning the hip hinge pattern (with proper lumbopelvic rhythm) first. Together, a better awareness of lumbopelvic rhythm (motor control), the ability to articulate the hips in a manner that maintains a neutral spine when picking up an object, and the ability to effectively use the hips to create a hinge pattern and lock the lumbar spine into a static and stable position allow better usage of the glutes and hamstrings as prime movers instead of stabilizers.

In other words, posterior chain development, particularly of the glute complex and hamstrings, is a critical component of effective lower body training for health, longevity, performance, and athletics. While we know that the posterior plays a major role in overall success (whether in terms of health or performance), this isn't to say that you should neglect training the anterior region of the body; quite the contrary.

Instead, you should have an optimal balance of posterior versus anterior chain training and choose exercises that fit individual goals, needs, and anthropometrics (limb length), as well as consistently allow for motor pattern improvement. (The execution of the hip hinge pattern needs consistent attention because becoming complacent may put you at risk of injury.)

While quad-dominant exercises are important and will certainly be covered in great depth, understanding how strength in the posterior regions of the body that support both local motion and the hip hinge pattern plays a key role in lower back integrity is important for any strength and conditioning professional. A baseline level of knowledge with regard to hip- and quad-dominant and abduction- and adduction-dominant movements is the starting point to create more balance through movement and to strategically include specific movements in your program design. This will give you the ability to do the following:

- *Assess limitations.* Since the human body is not completely symmetrical, neither is the ratio of strength between limbs. The ability to identify areas of opportunity for training focus and to select exercises based on those limitations is important for health and strength improvement. For instance, if an individual has a one-rep max front squat that is close to their one-rep max deadlift, that individual is limited in terms of posterior chain recruitment and maximal strength. Programming variations can then be included that address limitations of the musculature that drives hip extension and hip abduction, which will balance out the ratio of strength between the posterior and anterior chains of the individual.
- *Create balance within program design specific to need.* Using the same example, offsetting the distribution of hip-dominant versus quad-dominant work in favor of the former will be important.
- *Address limitations related to job descriptions.* If we know an individual works a desk job and is sitting for extended periods, it will make sense to counter these anatomical positions (i.e., more hip-dominant patterns). The overwhelming majority of individuals will present common posture maladies. We counter these maladies with movements that pull people into healthier postures.

Table 2.1 provides examples of what quad-dominant, hip-dominant, hip adduction, and hip abduction movement patterns look like in terms of exercise selection to give you a better understanding of what these terms mean and how they could play out within a training program.

Table 2.1 Movement Pattern Examples

Hip-dominant	Quad-dominant	Hip abduction	Hip adduction
Sumo stance deadlift	Front squat	Landmine lateral squat	Adduction machine
Barbell Romanian deadlift	Goblet squat	Abduction machine	Banded adduction
Trap bar Romanian deadlift	Dumbbell forward lunge	X-band walk	Side-lying adduction
Glute bridge	Air squat	Fire hydrant	Standing hip adduction with a band

PRIORITIZING HIP- VERSUS QUAD-DOMINANT MOVEMENT PATTERNS

It's fairly well established in the strength training community that training the musculature of the glute complex and hamstrings provides a noteworthy return on investment in terms of health (in particular lower back health), longevity, and performance. The question is, how do we distribute movements within a training program to prioritize hip-dominant patterns over quad-dominant patterns? While you can find studies on the connection between glute strength and reduction of lower back pain, throwing out a blanket number for optimal ratio of hip- versus quad-dominant patterns would disregard bioindividuality. However, anecdotally speaking, a large majority of clients with whom I work have incurred great success when we favor the posterior chain in our exercise selection. So what does this mean, exactly?

I have found that a ratio of 2:1 hip-dominant versus quad-dominant exercises can have a profound effect on individuals who have desk jobs or sit for the majority of the day. Moreover, as the incidence of lower back disorders rises, we know that strengthening the supporting musculature of the glutes and hamstrings can help create awareness of lumbopelvic rhythm, and using hinging patterns in the gym and in everyday life can reduce undue stress on the lumbar spine. These facts point toward prioritizing more hip-dominant patterns, but of course one size never fits all, and optimal ratios should be determined on a case-by-case basis.

Table 2.2 Sample Training Sessions With 2:1 Hip- Versus Quad-Dominant Ratio

Exercise	Sets	Reps	Rest
Training session 1			
Box squat	5	5	120 sec
Trap bar Romanian deadlift	4	8-10	90 sec
Goblet squat	3	12-15	60 sec
Back raise	3	30	60 sec
Training session 2			
Sumo stance rack deadlift	Build in weight over 9 sets	1RM	180 sec
Glute-ham raise	4	8-10	90 sec
Dumbbell reverse lunge	3	8-10 each side	60 sec
Cable pull-through	4	15	60 sec

As an example of this 2:1 ratio, table 2.2 shows two sample training sessions for the lower body that focus more on hip-dominant patterns but still include work for the anterior chain and quadriceps development.

One of the more difficult aspects of achieving this 2:1 ratio is selecting exercises that match your goals. People often get "paralysis by analysis" from the sheer number of exercise variations at their disposal; however, this book is intended to help you zero in on tried-and-true exercises to allow you to arrive at your desired result of performance and longevity. With that said, knowing how to make substitutions based on what you have at your disposal is important. If you don't have access to a full commercial gym or complex equipment, the simplicity of dumbbells, a landmine, and bands can provide positive training effects. Table 2.3 provides some exercise examples. The number of options is virtually unlimited, even with minimal equipment.

Table 2.3 Options for Bilateral and Unilateral Hip- and Quad-Dominant Exercises Using Simple Equipment

Quad-dominant exercise options		Hip-dominant exercise options	
Bilateral	**Unilateral**	**Bilateral**	**Unilateral**
Front squat	Forward lunge	Trap bar Romanian deadlift	Barbell single-leg Romanian deadlift
1-1/4 front squat	Barbell front rack reverse lunge	Sumo deadlift	Single-leg back raise
Anderson front squat	Dumbbell split squat	Rack deadlift	Single-leg glute hip thrust
Front squat to pins	Box step-up	Glute hip thrust	Single-leg Romanian deadlift
Front box squat	Walking lunge	Reverse band Romanian deadlift	Dumbbell single-leg Romanian deadlift
Air squat	Goblet reverse lunge	Banded pull-through	Single-leg banded hamstring curl
Dumbbell goblet squat	Dumbbell reverse lunge	Dumbbell Romanian deadlift	Single-leg landmine Romanian deadlift
Goblet box squat	Landmine lateral squat	Glute bridge	
Double kettlebell box squat		Double-leg banded hamstring curl	
Banded air squat			

While the list of exercise variations for the lower body is extensive, a better option is focusing on the route of each movement pattern first—this promotes better movement competency and allows motor patterns to be ingrained before you attempt any of these movement progressions. The beauty of these movement patterns is that they do not require any specialized equipment; significant progress can be made with basic items. For beginner and novice individuals, movement competency is paramount to achieving long-lasting results and, most importantly, longevity in the resistance training game. In fact, it is the successful foundation to build upon with load and exercise variations that are higher up on the movement hierarchy pyramid.

Chapter 3

Go Beyond the Basics

It's no secret that training big core lifts like the front squat and sumo stance deadlift will produce delayed training effects; more importantly, because the range of motion (ROM) is significant with these lifts, the hormonal response in the body is also significant. We are going to address hormonal response and cover a variety of strength training methods, including the repeated effort method, the maximal effort (ME) method, the submaximal effort method, and the dynamic effort (DE) method, as well as general physical preparedness (GPP) work. You will see throughout this book that being aware of the adaptations that take place from each method, the demand on the nervous system from each method, and the overall goal for each method is critical to designing effective training programs that are balanced and thorough.

It's common for individuals to attempt the "next best thing" instead of adhering to tried-and-true methods that have been around for decades. It's also important to note that not all methods have the same intent and each method has a specific place and desired stimulus—you will notice how synergy can be created by using opposing methods. The benefits of blending opposing methods are twofold: (1) variability in bar velocity (bar speed), which utilizes both the force and velocity components of the force-velocity curve to create different training effects and neurological adaptations (Haff and Bompa 2009); and (2) the ability to prevent overtraining. Favoring one method over others presents challenges in terms of motor recruitment and, more importantly, risks overuse injuries and overtraining (e.g., performing ME training too often only utilizes the force component of strength training and does not present differing demands on the CNS). In short, each method described will serve a specific and unique purpose for you, and while not all methods need to

The Force-Velocity Curve

When different strength development methods are used, there is more potential for altering the force-velocity curve. The force-velocity curve examines the interactions between force and velocity and suggests there is an inverse relationship: when external resistance increases, movement velocity decreases (maximal effort work); and when external resistance decreases, movement velocity increases (Haff and Bompa 2009). See figure for an example of the force-velocity curve.

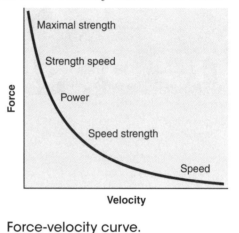

Force-velocity curve.

be used simultaneously, you will learn how to balance your plan of attack by working both ends of the force-velocity curve.

HORMONAL RESPONSES OF STRENGTH TRAINING

The benefits of effective lower limb training extend to optimal hormone production because the lower body represents the largest muscle groups in the body that signal the growth hormone insulin-like growth factor 1 (IGF-1) and serum testosterone. It's been widely established that long-term heavy resistance training can bring about significant increases of muscle size, strength, and power. These increases can boost hormonal interactions, and the type of exercise is a major player in how big the hormonal response is. Because heavy compound movements like squats and deadlifts require high levels of motor-unit recruitment, they activate androgen receptors for anabolic hormones such as testosterone. The inflammatory response to skeletal muscle damage causes remodeling to take place and consequently new growth to occur. Moreover, long-term training effects from heavy lower body resistance exercises can result in adaptations in the endocrine system, thus creating an environment in the human body that is suited for transport of anabolic hormones.

Therefore, heavy resistance training is a requisite for creating an anabolic environment in the human body that is more capable of gaining lean tissue; and gains in lean tissue are closely related to gains in maximal strength because cell size and volume are synonymous with improved motor-unit recruitment (Kraemer, Vingren, and Spiering 2016).

While you don't need to be an exercise physiologist to understand the positive effect strength training produces with regard to anabolic (muscle-building) hormones, it is important to have a baseline level of knowledge about the training effects of lower body training. It seems logical that the largest muscles in the human body are going to facilitate spikes in hormones that involve building strength and muscle mass.

There are a couple things to consider in addition to the roles of IGF-1, growth hormone, testosterone, and insulin. The first thing is your training age or the total amount of time you've spent performing resistance training because this can dictate improvements that take place from a neural standpoint; there is more to the picture than just hormonal response. For instance, it is common for beginners just starting strength training to see improvement in strength before seeing large gains in muscle hypertrophy. Beginner-level individuals may add 40 to 50 pounds (18 to 23 kg) to their squat and deadlift in as little as 16 weeks owing to neural adaptations that take place upon initial exposure to strength training.

Over the course of your first 8 to 12 weeks of a strength training program, you typically see a much faster rate of strength improvement due to direct factors relating to the nervous system, such as:

- Increased neural drive
- Increased neural coordination
- Increased motor-unit synchronization

These physiological changes (among many others) allow a beginner to recruit more high-threshold motor units, leading to an increase in type II muscle fiber activation. Not only can an individual recruit more high-threshold motor units, but the firing rate (rate coding) may also become more synchronous with other high-threshold motor units, which will affect the onset of discharge and therefore improve the rate of force development (RFD). This increase in RFD means an athlete requires a shorter time to reach maximal force (this helps translate to explosive movements). After the initial 8 to 12 weeks, increase in muscle hypertrophy becomes a more important factor, further increasing maximal strength (Schoenfeld 2021). In short, while strength training has positive effects on anabolic hormone production, this is only one piece of the puzzle; it is important to understand that this process is multifaceted and very much dictated by your overall training experience (or lack of experience).

STRENGTH TRAINING AND ITS RELATION TO OTHER BIOMOTOR ABILITIES

Before we delve into the various methods of strength development, it is important to understand what strength is. Although one can read about strength in just about any exercise physiology book, let's review a few key definitions first and see how and why strength is relevant to your training program. It's important to note that strength provides the basis for success across multiple modalities, as well as increased resiliency and longevity; and it connects to every biomotor ability (see figure 3.1).

There is no question that strength is the ultimate biomotor ability and carries over to improvements in other important fitness characteristics such as speed, power, and muscle endurance. So even if the goal isn't necessarily to improve upon maximal strength (increasing your one-rep max squat), there are still connections between maximal strength and other abilities such as strength endurance. For example, if your one-rep max squat increases, it's likely that your five-rep max will too.

By definition, strength is the ability of a given muscle or muscle group to generate force (Haff and Bompa 2009). While there are a number of scenarios for strength to be manifested, the training methods presented later in this chapter will help provide context around how strength is developed, its classifications, and specific guidelines on how to develop each type of strength. The exercises and training programs provided later in this book will also include appropriate rep schemes that coincide with these methods. Different strength methods all contribute to increasing

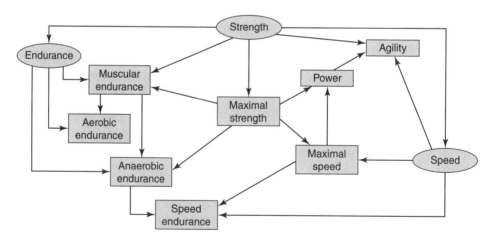

Figure 3.1 Interaction of biomotor abilities and various aspects of sports performance.

Reprinted by permission from T. Bompa and C.A. Buzzichelli, *Periodization: Theory and Methodology of Training*, 6th ed. (Champaign, IL: Human Kinetics, 2019), 231.

strength qualities, but establishing a baseline level of maximal strength (assuming you have built efficient movement patterns with a given lift) will ensure that all qualities are increasing commensurately. Each strength method has a specific intent and specific parameters that are important when using a concurrent (training multiple biomotor abilities within the same week of training) form of training.

Also, understanding the adaptations that take place from various forms of strength training helps ensure that your training program will promote balanced strength development. Maximal force or velocity of a muscle or a muscle group can be expressed in other biomotor abilities like speed and endurance. We hear many individuals say things like "I'm not concerned with gaining maximal strength" simply because they are not yet educated in the connection between maximal strength and nearly every other biomotor ability.

Now that we've established that maximal strength plays a key role in the strength development of other biomotor abilities, it is important for you to understand its other advantages, which may not be obvious to the untrained eye:

- *Synergy of strength modalities.* It's important to know the differences between strength training methods and how they blend together in a successful training plan. With this in mind, this book will use a variety of strength training measures that look to improve different components of strength at different locations on the force-velocity curve (maximal force versus maximal velocity). This allows you to effectively create balance within a training plan and prevent overtraining.

- *Improvement of strength limitations.* As Louie Simmons says, "You're only as strong as your weakest link." This holds true with developing lower body strength. A consistent attack on limitations with a wide variety of special exercises will prevent weak links from destabilizing your training and is instrumental to your lower body training success (Simmons 2015). You cannot effectively build a base of strength if you're neglecting general strength measures (i.e., unilateral work, which not only allows you to consistently address your limitations but sets up success with other modalities such as maximal strength work).

- *Avoiding accommodation or adapting to a repetitive stimulus.* The biological law of accommodation states that constant exposure to the same stimulus results in detraining. In order to prevent accommodation, exercise selection and volume prescriptions should be adjusted regularly (Simmons 2015). We know the body thrives on variability in order to continue to make progress, and this variability will come by way of varying exercise selection while still programming the essential foundational patterns of squatting, lunging, and hip hinging.

- *Improving motor-unit recruitment as it relates to strength training.* Maximal strength work has the ability to recruit and use higher-threshold motor units.

In short, having a firm grasp on the methods and their overall goals will be instrumental in creating better synergy, adaptations, and improvement of limitations. It is clear that heavy lower body resistance training has massive returns on investment with regard to improving maximal strength, which has strong ties to performance, but understanding the endocrinology of multijoint training is a key factor in creating an anabolic environment in the human body. You need to make the connection that growth can only occur in an optimal stress environment. Detraining can also occur if you undergo doses of heavy resistance training that are too *high*. For example, stress levels that are too high (by way of a training session being too long in duration or simply using high-intensity measures too frequently in one's program design) can increase catabolic hormones such as cortisol that may override anabolic hormones, thus delaying positive training adaptations or eventually leading to central fatigue. In short, how you manage stress within the training session affects the success of your training; there is a fine line between too much volume, intensity, or frequency and not enough stress to induce positive training adaptations.

STRENGTH TRAINING METHODS

Now that we've examined the various qualities of strength training, we'll dive into the training methods, in order of importance. These methods will be used in the programs provided in part III of the book. However, with any training method comes a number of caveats. For instance, the ME method is an incredibly effective method to build absolute strength, but it may simply be out of alignment if you're not advanced in terms of training age, training history, and motor control with bilateral movements such as the squat and deadlift. The old adage "one must learn to crawl before one can walk" rings true with strength training, and the foundation of strength training is built with "general strength" measures such as unilateral exercises. The methods are therefore presented in the order of which will have the largest effect on your current training state fastest. Later in this book, we'll highlight exercise variations and how those variations are sequenced with a training plan specifically geared at developing lower limb strength. Keep in mind that while this book is designed to improve your knowledge and understanding of optimal lower body programming, the same logic, tenets, and methods can be applied when programming for the upper body.

General Physical Preparedness Work

The term *general physical preparedness* (GPP) gets thrown around quite a bit—many coaches claim that the goal of their program is to develop GPP, yet many of these same coaches don't use measures that actually develop it. Throwing heavy deadlifts into a workout if you are already lacking in the strength department won't develop GPP and will likely get you hurt. We are talking about building your foundation. This is something that should take precedence in any programming—if you cannot pull a sled or carry two heavy kettlebells without having to rest excessively between sets, then higher-skill work like ME squats or deadlifts isn't a smart move. The Russians had a GPP plan for all of their athletes called the "rule of three" that they employed for three years in the early stages of training *before* specialization took place. Yup, you read that right. Why is this relevant to your training programs? If the Russians were smart enough to build their athletes' foundations first, then maybe this is something you should consider. More importantly, all of the training goals expressed by most people (*look better, feel better, get stronger, have fun*) can be addressed with GPP measures.

Improving maximal strength indirectly connects to qualities of strength endurance, although the two strengths could not be further from each other. Using measures like sled drags, we can effectively improve aerobic capacity and oxidative qualities of the musculature of the hips, hamstrings, and calves, as well as bridge the gap between ME and DE training sessions. Think of the sled as an intermediary to improve strength qualities with only a small cost on the nervous and muscular systems due to the fact there is zero axial loading. Moreover, the sled also will improve the oxidative quality of fast-twitch muscle fibers.

Fast-twitch type II muscle fibers have an aerobic as well as anaerobic ability, which strengthens the connection between maximal and submaximal strength development and strength endurance. Unfortunately, sled work is less common and accessible at a commercial gym, but times have changed and many folks are now investing in their own home gyms. The sled is an expensive training tool that is the difference maker between reasonable gains and exceptional gains—it really is that powerful. The sled may be one of the most valuable training tools we have available, and at less than 120 dollars it is cost-effective.

The sled is a mainstay in effective program design and can be used for strengthening as well as restoration. In addition, we can effectively train all three energy systems with the sled, and while this book is geared more toward strength development than it is conditioning, it would be foolish to not mention the benefits that the sled provides for both strength and conditioning that are different from those of any other training modality.

One can perform both short and long intervals of work with this tool, making it quite versatile. In the programs presented in part III of the book, schemes will be presented for programming sled work optimally and logically so it is building upon other modalities such as ME work. Moreover, sled work is a great way to unload the body and expedite recovery. And building upon our unilateral versus bilateral debate, the sled in essence is a unilateral training modality where both legs and arms work contralaterally, allowing you to continuously address asymmetries. Additionally, because the arms and legs are working in a contralateral fashion comparable to that of a normal walking gait, the sled can actually improve the most basic human function of local motion.

GPP is a huge aspect of any successful strength and conditioning program. Although GPP is often an afterthought and usually traded for "sexier modalities" like squats or deadlifts, the use of tools like the sled on a regular basis as well as high-volume band work to improve connective tissue quality and strengthen tendons can be the catalyst for longevity and consistency as far as strength and hypertrophy gains are concerned. And while this work is prescribed more anecdotally, with no peer-reviewed research to support its efficacy, it makes complete sense given the physiology of how tendons work. The storage of kinetic energy takes place in the series elastic component (SEC), the musculotendinous unit within our tendons, which will also be addressed in parts II and III where plyometrics are employed to improve explosive strength qualities. The rapid nature of accommodating resistance (AR) band exercises and the band's ability to be executed with rapid movement can increase the storage of kinetic energy within tendons (Potach and Chu 2016). Therefore, the makeup of high-volume, rapid band exercises supports the notion that tendon quality and stiffness can be improved in this manner. In fact, Westside Barbell, the "strongest gym in the world" that we discussed previously, relies heavily on higher-volume band exercises such as leg curls and pushdowns to prevent soft-tissue injuries when pushing loads with maximal weights. The good news is that this band work can be done just about anywhere with a few inexpensive bands on hand, making this option great for the home gym. Additionally, for the amount of time that's needed for this work on a daily basis (5 to 10 minutes), the return on investment is sizable.

To recap, building a base of fitness is done most effectively with measures that would be considered "general" in nature, like single-joint exercises performed in typical hypertrophy and strength endurance schemes or sled drag variations that provide a high volume of work with little cost on the nervous and muscular systems. However, let's not forget that while incurring tissue breakdown and rebuilding is part of gaining new muscle mass, there must be a way to bridge the gap and expedite recovery—you're only as good as your ability to recover between sessions. This is best accomplished with tools such as a sled and bands, which both provide unique benefits that go beyond strength qualities. So if your training plan is going to be complete, modalities like sled drags and high-volume band exercises are a must. These variations are included in the training programs provided in part III.

Repeated Effort Method

The repeated effort method is a premier method of improving muscular imbalance and muscular hypertrophy and providing rehabilitative or prehabilitative work to ensure you're constantly improving symmetry. This work is done through single-joint exercises and isolation work to target musculature limitations. It's important to prioritize unilateral assistance exercises because you can dedicate time to improving limitations, and classic lifts such as the squat, press, and deadlift will improve through establishing symmetry and strength in lagging muscle groups. Because unilateral exercises are less demanding on the nervous system, you are able to add volume and frequency with the overall objective of improving deficiencies. The volume of assistance exercises can be pushed to high levels and align with your training age and needs quite well with less risk. Moreover, people often fail to take inventory of where they struggle the most and experiment with exercises that will potentially help improve their limiting factors. This is what assistance exercises are for—to strategically improve limitations in a muscle or muscle group that may be holding one back, or worse, increasing their risk of injury in the future. A simple example of this is the glutes, which extend the hips and abduct and externally rotate the legs. They are therefore responsible for the finishing, hip extension–based portions of the squat and deadlift. Performing exercises that duplicate these actions is key. The Romanian deadlift (RDL) and the glute hip thrust are two excellent choices to build glute strength around hip extension movements.

Of course, improving performance is important to many individuals, but many people tend to have the primary goal of improving body composition. Luckily, assistance exercise work can be instrumental in helping add lean muscle mass because the 8- to 12-rep range will facilitate muscular hypertrophy (also known as sarcoplasmic hypertrophy), which is an increase in the volume of sarcoplasmic fluid in the muscle cell with no actual increase in muscular strength—envision the "muscle pump" you get after doing three sets of biceps curls (French 2016). In this case, time under tension will be significantly higher than for your max effort, and DE work as the objective is quite different in terms of strength development. (Hypertrophy work prioritizes time under tension, whereas DE work prioritizes bar velocity to improve RFD.) The ultimate goal here is to improve and isolate lagging muscle groups, so single-joint exercises like split squats, single-leg RDLs, and glute hip thrust variations are pillars of effective lower body program design.

Benefits of Prioritizing Assistance Exercises

The benefits of prioritizing assistance exercises (roughly 80 percent of your training volume in a given session) are understated. Of course, it's much sexier to squat with a barbell than it is to split squat with two dumbbells, but the latter allows you to execute higher volumes of work with less chance of compensation and will carry over to improve your squat numbers through improved motor-neuron synchronization. The benefits of prioritization are the following:

Focuses Lagging Muscle Groups

In an effort to target where you may be lacking, we can add a high volume of work without the risk of exacerbating compensation patterns—this will carry over to bigger movements like squats and deadlifts by improving muscle function and coordination with other muscles.

Safely Creates Higher Volume Through Unilateral Movements

It is much safer to push the volume of a unilateral movement like a split squat than a bilateral movement like a back squat. Pushing the volume on compound movements carries inherent risks of overuse injury and creating compensation patterns—with heavy, high-rep bilateral work, there will almost always be a breakdown in the chain as fatigue sets in. This can exacerbate your current asymmetries and set you up for injury instead of making actual improvements.

Increases the Time Under Tension

Unilateral work requires less skill and neural demand, so we can increase loading and volume commensurately, thereby increasing time under tension. This leads to increasing muscular hypertrophy. Sarcoplasmic hypertrophy is a product of time under tension, unlike maximal strength development, where time under tension is much lower.

Improves Bilateral Movement Motor Control and Performance

To improve bilateral movements like squats, pulls, and Olympic lifts, you have to have a continuous focus on isolating the areas where you are weakest. For many, something as simple as adding more direct posterior chain work is all it takes to produce noticeable gains in all of the previously mentioned lifts (glute hip thrusts, back raises, and RDL variations) and is a great vehicle to improve lifts where the posterior chain predominates, such as squats, deadlifts, and even the Olympic lifts.

Reduces the Risk of Injury

Assistance exercise work can effectively reduce the risk of injury as well as rehabilitate current injuries. Advanced individuals must be constantly assessing where they may be most limited; otherwise they risk eventually incurring a setback or even detraining effects. Strategically isolating weak muscle groups with unilateral exercises can bring someone back from injury as well as prevent future injuries.

Maximal Effort Method

The ME method is considered the superior method of improving both intramuscular and intermuscular coordination; the muscles and CNS adapt only to the load placed upon them, and this method brings forth the greatest strength gains (Zatsiorsky, Kraemer, and Fry 2021). With that said, what is meant by "maximal" can span a number of scenarios, making the ME method a polarizing topic to say the least. Is training maximally done with multiple repetitions such as a two-, three-, or even five-rep max? Or are we talking about simply loading the bar with as much weight as one can move for one repetition? In this book, we are referring to maximal tension with the heaviest load for one repetition. The ME method here is lifting a maximal load for one repetition performed with bilateral movements such as squat, deadlift, and press variations. These variations are included in the training programs provided in part III.

The adaptations occur in both intermuscular and intramuscular coordination—in essence improving both the ability of muscles to fire in synchronicity with one another and motor patterns. The ME method brings forth the greatest gains in maximal strength with the most amount of motor units activated (Zatsiorsky, Kraemer, and Fry 2021) and has the highest-intensity strength measure (maximum load/resistance for one repetition) but lowest-volume bilateral training measure (intensity and volume should not intersect with this method) (Simmons 2015).

As previously mentioned, there are connections between maximal strength and other biomotor abilities like strength endurance, but we must first consider if the ME method can fit into your training plan, allowing you to arrive at optimal results and a favorable risk-versus-reward ratio. Exercise variations should be rotated *weekly* to reduce risk of injury and to identify variations that are anthropometrically most suited to the individual. Also, individuals using this method should be fully comfortable building to one-rep maximum with any foundational movement pattern such as a box squat or a floor press. Another safety note is that this method requires the use of a spotter every time.

While this method does come with a stigma of being dangerous and is not recommended for beginner or even intermediate individuals, it's only dangerous if the individual has not learned how to properly perform the big lifts. Not having learned proper motor patterns can be a detriment with any method, but it's certainly not prudent to imagine working with maximal loads without the proper movement patterns enforced first. However, there are certainly other methods that will be a better match for novices.

Submaximal Effort Method

The submaximal effort method differs from the ME method in the number of repetitions executed, not necessarily the level of effort. While the ME method results in the highest levels of motor-unit recruitment, the submaximal effort method still results in high levels of motor-unit recruitment that correspond with the size principle—recruitment order is determined by the load placed upon the body; as the relative load increases across multiple repetitions, large motor units will be recruited (Zatsiorsky, Kraemer, and Fry 2021). With that said, the adaptations with this method will be different from those with the ME method; however, a key takeaway is that this method is optimal for individuals who have less experience. This is because the emphasis is on building motor patterns with more exposure to lighter loads. Individuals will not typically be asked to go to one-rep maximum if they are still learning how to move with a given pattern. Performing a multiple-rep max with a bilateral movement such as a squat variation technically constitutes submaximal work—remember that true ME work is trained with a maximum singular effort.

The adaptations for this method are intermuscular and intramuscular coordination—in essence improving both the ability of muscles to fire in synchronicity with one another and motor patterns. Also, time under tension is higher and results in more hypertrophic adaptations. The submaximal effort method presents moderate-intensity, moderate-volume measure—it's recommended that you do not attempt to ramp up to the same degree one would expect with a method like the repeated effort method. Exercise variations should be rotated every two to three weeks to allow time to ingrain good motor patterns.

In short, the logic behind the submaximal effort method is twofold: (1) improve motor patterns with bigger bilateral movements—this is critical for newer individuals before attempting to progress to a method such as the ME method; and (2) incur higher bouts of volume with bigger lifts. Remember, you will still incur the largest volume with the repeated effort method and smaller unilateral exercises, but that's not to say that including heavier multiple-rep maxes with bilateral movements does not have a place in your training plan. You must be mindful of proper volume prescriptions and how this method synergizes with other methods, which will play out optimally in the programs in part III.

Dynamic Effort Method

The DE method is used not to increase maximal strength but only to improve the RFD and explosive strength (Zatsiorsky, Kraemer, and Fry 2021). Working harder is often associated with making more gains in the gym, but I'd urge you to consider working smarter. The different methods introduced here will allow you to create a more well-rounded training plan that covers all bases in terms of special strength development. The DE method works with lighter loads and emphasizes bar velocity; only working with submaximal or maximal loads does not offer the benefits of dedicating time to work on bar velocity or power such as with the DE method. Oftentimes people associate power training with the Olympic lifts, and while there is certainly a power component to the Olympic lifts, for many the Olympic lifts are not practical as they require years of experience and coaching from a qualified coach. Instead, you can arrive at the same improvements in RFD, in this case speed strength, by using the DE method without having to learn the snatch or clean and jerk. Again, the focus is on bar velocity against intermediate resistance, which will provide better results than simply using ME or submaximal effort training alone.

The DE method is integral for improving RFD and explosive strength. (We'll learn more about explosive strength work via plyometrics in parts II and III.) In fact, there are a number of peer-reviewed studies that support the efficacy of speed training (DE training) in terms of motor-unit recruitment, improving fast-twitch type II muscle fibers, and improving the elastic abilities of muscles and tendons (Cormie, McGuigan, and Newton 2011). Because of this, it is prudent to include such training in a well-rounded training plan. Even if your goal is to gain lean muscle mass, this method will provide a synergistic effect when used with other methods such as the ME method. The volume in the DE method is significantly higher than that of the ME method, so together the two methods correspond with each other to optimize gains in both speed strength and strength speed and to prevent overtraining. On your DE training days, the inclusion of explosive strength work via plyometrics allows you to add a vital component of improving RFD as well as maintaining type II fibers, which is particularly beneficial to aging individuals. In short, when methods like the ME and DE methods are used in conjunction with each other in the same week of training, it creates a symbiotic relationship between methods that, in essence, oppose but blend well with one another. The DE and ME methods are different but present similar demands on the CNS.

Furthermore, this method gives an advantage when trying to mimic the specificity of a sport. For instance, American football plays last between four and seven seconds, with 45 to 60 seconds of rest between plays. You can easily replicate this pattern by using the box squat, performing eight triples every 45 to 60 seconds. This trains the ability of the aerobic system to replenish high-energy phosphates, which is critical for success in a sport like American football; while this sport draws largely on the anaerobic adenosine triphosphate–phosphocreatine (ATP-PC) system, there is a component of replenishing ATP aerobically since the athlete does not receive full recovery between efforts. Moreover, this work carries over to other sports such as ice or field hockey or soccer where explosive bursts of movement are needed. In this case, the demands can be aligned with the time domains of each sport allowing an athlete to effectively train specificity that will have a real-world carryover to their sport.

The adaptations for this method are intermuscular and intramuscular coordination, in essence improving both the ability of muscles to fire in synchronicity with one another and motor patterns. The DE method presents a high-intensity, moderate-volume measure—the focus is on bar velocity and perfect technique, not maximal loading. Exercise variations should be rotated every three weeks to allow for time to ingrain good motor patterns and increase loading each subsequent week. Furthermore, the DE method will help maintain type II fibers that deteriorate with age (Potach and Chu 2016). Lastly, to fully reap the benefits of the DE method, using AR is recommended. Even if you are not an athlete or do not care about becoming more explosive, the DE method has a place within your program. Again, the adaptations are different from those of the other methods, which creates favorable circumstances.

Explosive Strength

While jumping is an integral part of improving explosive strength for athletics, it has value in terms of physiology and type II muscle fibers

Optimal Volume Prescriptions for Training Methods

This chapter would not be complete without discussing optimal volume recommendations for all methods. The following table shows optimal Olympic weightlifting rep ranges used for training. Known as Prilepin's Chart, it was created by A.S. Prilepin, a Soviet-era sports scientist who reviewed the training journals of thousands of weightlifting athletes. It is meant to portray the optimal number of reps per set and total rep count (volume) for power training required for the Olympic lifts (the snatch and the clean and jerk).

Percent of 1RM	Approximate number of repetitions	Optimal number of reps	Total range
40%	4-8	36	30-50
50%	3-6	30	18-30
60%	3-6	24	18-30
70%	3-6	18	12-24
80%	2-4	15	10-20
90+%	1-2	4-10	1-10

Adapted from Prilepin's Chart, A.S. Prilepin.

This chart has stood the test of time, and I've used it extensively over the last decade. Of course, a guide is just that, a guide, and never one-size-fits-all, but this chart is a great starting point when attempting to arrive at optimal volume with the ME, submaximal effort, and DE methods.

even for people who simply want to look and feel better and hit new personal records from time to time. For those who don't have any interest in athletic competition or powerlifting, the question comes down to determining proper volume prescriptions and plyometric variations. In terms of programming for general fitness, performing 20 to 25 jumps twice a week is more than sufficient to prime the sympathetic nervous system prior to a training session or as a stand-alone movement for explosive strength work. The benefits span beyond improving power and RFD because we know that type II fibers deteriorate as folks age— plyometrics can be a powerful catalyst for maintaining those type II fibers, and the return on a small investment of time is significant (Potach and Chu 2016).

For athletes, on the other hand, plyometrics can certainly serve as a permanent fixture in multiple sessions each week in which programmed volume is higher and the skill requisite of variations can be higher. (This is not always the case because the basic variations are still vital.) Of course, this would need to be specific to the individual based on their training age, the bioenergetics of their chosen sport, and their training history (to include proper ability for jumping and landing mechanics).

When used correctly, plyometric training has been shown to improve the production of muscle force and power, so not only will regular plyometric work help with the overall goal of body composition, but it will also improve performance. Moreover, since we know the sympathetic nervous system's fight-or-flight response and post-activation potentiation last roughly five to eight minutes, we can effectively use some form of plyometrics to serve as a proper warm-up tool and prime the CNS for a maximal lift that requires high levels of motor-unit recruitment.

Choosing variations doesn't have to be overly complicated. A few variations that are low in skill requisite and impact are shown in table 3.1.

Table 3.1 Lower-Skill and Low-Impact Plyometric Variations

Plyometric variation	Sets	Reps	Rest
Seated dynamic vertical jump	6	3	45-60 sec
Seated dynamic box jump	6	3	45-60 sec
Dumbbell squat jump + box jump	6	2	60 sec
Trap bar jump	5	4	60 sec

With these variations it would be easy to increase or decrease difficulty based on individual needs by simply modifying the jump height or adding resistance, but if you are not comfortable jumping and landing, there are other available options such as static isometrics that have carryover and training effects similar to those of dynamic plyometrics.

In short, you will find that it is advantageous to have many tools in your toolbox as far as strength training is concerned, and simply working "hard" doesn't mean results are guaranteed. Instead, it's best to work smarter and understand the stress cycle the body goes through with the ebbs and flows of high-intensity training—this is a major reason why we've talked about other measures (repeated effort method and GPP work) that act as a bridge between your more demanding training sessions.

ADDITIONAL TRAINING TOOLS

Training for strength is comparable to building a house where each tool has a very specific focus and role. Tools such as cluster sets, accommodating resistance, reverse bands, sleds, barbells, kettlebells, dumbbells, or specialized machines all help an individual arrive at their desired result. Much like building a house, more tools in your toolbox will allow you to complete the task faster and more efficiently.

Cluster Sets

Using intraset rest or "clusters" is hardly a new concept. In fact, Olympic lifters use clusters regularly, some without even knowing it. Cluster training allows for small bouts of rest (10 to 20 seconds) in between reps to provide recovery and avoid the movement deterioration that would normally occur during a straight set with appreciable loading. In *Supertraining*, cluster training is categorized two ways: (1) *extensive clustering*, which involves four to six repetitions at four- to six-rep max with 10-second rest intervals between each cluster; and (2) *intensive clustering* with four to six total reps performed one repetition at a time at between 75 and 90 percent of one-rep max, with about 20 seconds of rest between repetitions (Verkhoshansky and Siff 2009). There is a place for both extensive and intensive clustering, and I've used both with great success. For purposes of hypertrophy, where the intent is longer time under tension, extensive clustering fits the bill and can be used with a myriad of movements that would normally cause high neural fatigue.

Cluster sets work quite well when used for general strength purposes. In part III of this book, I've applied cluster work in hypertrophy, strength, and athletic performance settings. Intermediate and even more advanced athletes can benefit from using intraset rest, and I'd even go so far as to say that for beginner athletes, having small bouts of rest between reps can help instill efficient movement patterns while minimizing the risk of mechanical breakdown or creating faulty motor patterns. Although it may seem that cluster sets are not necessary for general fitness, much like any other method we use, they are a tool that can spark some new progress. Cluster sets are a staple in my own personal programming and in my programming for my clients. Here are some reasons why it may be prudent to use clusters:

- Increased time under tension
- Improved movement patterns
- Increased neural drive with heavier loading
- Efficient use of time

Using cluster sets for the squat or other bilateral movements can be quite effective in improving your ability to perform higher amounts of volume with heavier loads. In the case of the squat, we prefer to opt for longer rest bouts of 15 to 25 seconds, depending on the objectives of your training session. Here are a few examples:

Front squat: 4 sets × 2.2.2 (15 sec) @ 80%. Rest 3 min.

1 set = perform 2 reps—rerack weight and rest 15 sec, followed by 2 reps + rest 15 sec + 2 reps + rest 3 min

Back squat: 4 sets × 3.2.1 (20 sec) @ 85%. Rest 3 min.

1 set = perform 3 reps—rerack weight and rest 20 sec, followed by 2 reps + rest 20 sec + 1 rep + rest 3 min

In short, cluster work is not only time-efficient but, more importantly, economical for increasing trainability of a given bilateral movement (squat, press, pulls) while simultaneously decreasing the risk of breakdown and thus the chance of overuse injury.

Accommodating Resistance

We alluded to the fact that using AR is optimal with the DE method, so let's explore what AR is and why it can be beneficial to your training plan. AR refers to the use of chains or bands to develop maximal tension throughout the full ROM, rather than at your weakest point. While there are a number of benefits to using AR, one of the most noteworthy is accommodating the strength curve, in which tension is highest where we are strongest and lowest where we are weakest (Simmons 2015). Here are a few key points when using AR:

Bands Versus Chains

The major difference between bands and chains is the phenomenon known as "overspeed eccentric." Put simply, in the case of a squat, bands actually pull you down in the lowering portion of your lift, increasing the amount of kinetic energy that is produced. Because of this, you are able to enhance reversal strength and your ability to absorb force, crucial to any sport. With chains, the overspeed eccentric is not present because the resistance does not stay consistent when an athlete is lowering the weight. Overall, using bands is particularly advantageous to strength athletes who want to become more explosive. These benefits can translate into cracking personal records in the big three.

- AR allows for greater accountability with bar speed compared to just straight weight—as tension increases through ROM, you are forced to accelerate through each repetition and not get complacent.
- AR coincides with the strength curve, meaning that your band tension will be highest where you are strongest (top of the movement) and lowest where you are weakest (bottom of the movement).
- The RFD provides more resistance without compromising bar speed with regard to the strength curve of a given movement (i.e., band tension is highest where you are strongest and vice versa).
- As weight increases, bar speed decreases. Maximal strength force is high, and velocity is low. AR gives you the ability to develop speed strength, whereas with simply adding straight weight, bar velocity will inevitably decline.
- AR teaches you how to absorb more force, which in turn allows you to become more powerful.
- Without bands or chains, bar deceleration is inevitable, and when bar speed is too slow, RFD simply cannot be developed. AR forces you to accelerate through full ROM, and becoming more explosive translates to becoming stronger!
- AR can also be used for ME work. The advantage here is that you will be able to use less straight weight, with overload occurring at the top of a given movement. As a result, external loading through ROM is lower, which equates to less breakdown and less delayed onset muscle soreness. For a movement like an ME rack deadlift,

where loading for some can reach supramaximal levels, using AR will reduce the amount of wear and tear compared to what would occur with just straight weight.

Reverse Bands

Reverse bands are the opposite of AR; bands are fixed to the top of the squat rack, and the load is lightest at the top and heaviest at the bottom as a given movement goes through eccentric ROM. (Think of the lowering phase of an RDL.) The benefits of using this method are improvements in neuromuscular efficiency and, more importantly, the ability to fine-tune and repattern foundational movements. In addition, being able to work with supramaximal loads at the top of each movement creates different scenarios from just working with straight weight—the degree to which you'll be able to exceed your one-rep max will depend on the thickness of the band you choose. Because you're able to work with supramaximal loads, this method tends to be quite demanding on the nervous system, particularly when used in true ME scenarios with big movements like the deadlift. However, in submaximal or repeated effort scenarios, you'll likely find you're able to maintain better position even with loads that exceed your current one-rep max. For the purposes of this book, though, we recommend the use of reverse bands not in an ME session but as an assistance exercise with a pattern like the RDL to reinforce (or rebuild) an effective hip hinge pattern (more on this in chapter 6). With that said, the reverse band method can also work quite well with repeated effort work and allow you to reinforce better movement patterns. Even if you approach loads where you would normally have some mechanical breakdown if you were using straight weight, the band will deload a percentage of the weight in the bottom position, thus allowing you to reinforce better motor patterns with less breakdown while still receiving the desired training effects.

Reverse bands are optimal when used for the following:

- *ME work:* one-repetition maximum (1RM)
- *Submaximal effort work:* 2-6RM
- *Repetition effort work:* 6- to 10-rep sets
- *Technique work:* Straight sets with moderately heavy loads of 80 to 85 percent of 1RM

These are the benefits of reverse bands:

- *Improved neuromuscular efficiency.* This is the ability of the nervous system to recruit the correct muscles to produce force.

- *Improved stability.* This is the ability of your body to stabilize and brace while achieving supramaximal loading at the end ROM.
- *Improved motor patterns.* Reverse bands deload a percentage of the weight at the bottom of a movement and allow you to in essence do the *opposite* of AR. Where with AR tension is highest where we are strongest (accommodating the strength curve), with reverse bands tension is highest where you are weakest.
- *Opportunity for technique work.* Reverse bands allow you to work with heavier loads with less chance of mechanical breakdown.
- *Hypertrophy.* If gaining lean mass is your goal, reverse bands work great with big movements so you can create situations with high amounts of metabolic stress but less mechanical breakdown.

In conclusion, the best part of using reverse bands is that they can serve a variety of purposes—maximal strength development, technique improvement, bodybuilding, and motor pattern refinement. The most critical aspect of this method is that it allows you to maximize trainability and decrease the risk of injury.

We've discussed multiple methods that build strength and learned that combining a variety of methods will not only improve your classic lifts such as the squat, bench press, and deadlift but also elicit gains in muscular hypertrophy. We've discussed the role maximal strength development has at the center of all strength training in terms of its connection to all biomotor abilities. Although many people are not concerned with improving their big lifts, understanding why maximal strength can have a role in someone's success makes it easy to build value in such methods as the ME method. It's also important to remember that using a variety of methods can help you avoid overuse injury and overtraining, and the diversity created with multiple methods in one's program design ensures that no stone is left unturned and that the training is varied enough to prevent accommodation.

Chapter 4

Set Realistic Training Goals

The results you obtain (or do not obtain) from your training are directly connected to setting realistic training goals. Oftentimes individuals set goals that are not within the realm of possibility, and many times through no fault of their own. Of course, it's common knowledge that beginners will be able to hit impressive personal records within a short period of time. On the other end of the spectrum, more advanced individuals are lucky to arrive at smaller improvements over the course of a year of training. As we touched upon in chapter 3, beginners are able to incur massive results within short periods as a result of neural adaptations that take place upon initial exposure to strength training. However, we know that no two individuals are the same, and creating reasonable training goals commensurate with their level of ability makes sense.

I'm going to highlight some very modest guidelines that you can apply to your own level of ability, but keep in mind that these guidelines are anecdotal in nature. Of course, it makes sense to establish concrete goals (which will be discussed in depth in this chapter) for strength, performance, and body composition improvements that resonate with the individual and align with their lifestyle, training age, training history, and needs. (The goals of a professional athlete will be very different from those of a soccer mom.) Moreover, you may be able to far exceed these expectations after applying the information found in this book because training smarter will always trump training harder. But overall, it's psychologically more prudent to set small goals that are achievable.

SMART GOALS

SMART is an acronym I learned a long time ago that describes what kind of goals to set:

- ***Specific.*** Establish a specific goal as it relates to your fitness. For instance, for a strength and power athlete this could mean making improvements to metrics like their vertical jump or one-rep max power clean, whereas someone training for general fitness may want to improve their waistline. The goal should be relevant to the individual.

- ***Measurable.*** Make sure you have the proper metrics to track throughout this process, whether that's a one-rep max squat or improving a 5K run. For example, you might start with a concise test and retest to accurately establish whether improvements have been made.

- ***Achievable.*** Set an achievable goal that is not only realistic within a given time frame but sets the stage for later success. Hitting this initial goal is important for keeping you engaged in the process. Oftentimes individuals set unrealistic goals, and when they fail to hit these goals, it derails their process. It's a better course of action to have a more reasonable goal.

- ***Relevant.*** This ties in with "specific" because the goal or goals should resonate with the individual and align with their current goals and lifestyle. As previously mentioned, if you're a professional athlete, your goals will likely relate to your sport, while a soccer mom may just want to have better energy levels and improve her body composition. For example, a goal of improving a one-rep max power clean would be out of alignment with a soccer mom's needs (assuming she is not competing in Olympic lifting). The goal must have bearing on the individual's reason for training.

- ***Time-bound.*** Set a date by which you're committed to reaching this goal. Having a time frame helps you to stay focused on the task at hand. Oftentimes I ask my own clients to commit to a date before starting. This date could be the date of a powerlifting meet, a time where they know they will be in front of others in a bathing suit, or whatever. Having that date in mind when they'll be held personally accountable helps facilitate compliance with the training plan.

All of these are critical aspects to setting realistic training goals that you can easily adopt as you start training or continue training so you're able to reap the benefits of your hard work and smash your goals!

What Metrics Matter?

Most experienced individuals who are interested in strength development would traditionally measure improvement in terms of their maximal load lifted in squat, bench press, and deadlift, but that's not to say that other metrics can't be considered. For metrics like body part measurements, there are no specific guidelines as to how much muscle mass one could gain within a 6- to 12-month training period, so establishing metrics and remeasuring every 16 weeks is a great place to start.

Body part measurements will allow you to objectively measure whether your training and nutrition are going in the right direction. Of course, I'd be remiss not to say that measurements are largely a marker of your success with your nutrition, and your nutrition will drive the results of your training whether you're looking to gain lean muscle mass or lose adipose tissue (fat stores).

Other strength metrics to keep track of include one-, two-, or three-rep maximums for your front or back squat; sumo stance, conventional, or trap bar deadlift; and bench press or floor press. I've listed multiple-rep maxes only for those who are not yet comfortable building to a maximum load, but keep in mind that multiple-rep maxes are not always a predictor of improvements in maximal strength. We've touched on the connections maximal strength has with every biomotor ability, but it's important to note that just because gains in maximal strength improve these other biomotor abilities, the inverse won't always be true (i.e., strength endurance improvement does not always equate to improving maximal strength). Moreover, keeping track of at least one conditioning metric would be good. To keep things simple, consider using a 10-minute air bike test for maximum calories as a great predictor of aerobic fitness or a 12-minute maximum distance run if conditioning performance is important to you.

Mindset training is often a forgotten aspect of coaching, and yet once we are able to shift someone's outlook on training so that they're able to see transformations happen before their very eyes, it's much easier for them to stay compliant and adopt habits that are sustainable for the rest of their lives.

REALISTIC GOALS FOR KEY LIFTS

With regard to what lifts are important to you, the suggestions in this book revolve around foundational movement patterns such as the squat, deadlift, and bench press, but these are not the only benchmarks to test and retest your progress. For instance, the squat for most is inherently a great movement, but there are plenty of people who cannot perform a full-depth squat (below parallel) efficiently. In other words, customizing the metric to your individual needs and authentic range of motion is important and will contribute to your longevity. With that said, the key performance indicator lifts provided in this book test absolute strength— the most load someone can move for one repetition regardless of their bodyweight.

Table 4.1 provides some basic guidelines that coincide with your level of ability for the squat, deadlift, and bench press. Not all of the

Table 4.1 Foundational Movement Pattern Improvements

Training experience	Repetition maximum (RM)	Recommended movements	1RM increase
<2 years	3-5RM	Squat variation: front box squat	Increase 10 lb (5 kg) every 16 weeks
		Deadlift variation: trap bar deadlift	Increase 15 lb (7 kg) every 16 weeks
		Bench press variation: floor press	Increase 5 lb (2 kg) every 16 weeks
2-4 years	2-4RM	Squat variation: box squat	Increase 7.5 lb (3.5 kg) every 16 weeks
		Deadlift variation: sumo stance deadlift	Increase 10 lb (5 kg) every 16 weeks
		Bench press variation: slight incline bench press	Increase 5 lb (2 kg) every 16 weeks
4+ years	1-2RM	Squat variation: front or back squat	Increase 5 lb (2 kg) every 16 weeks
		Deadlift variation: conventional rack deadlift	Increase 7.5 lb (3.5 kg) every 16 weeks
		Bench press variation: medium-grip bench press	Increase 2.5 lb (1 kg) every 16 weeks

exercise variations listed in table 4.1 are included in this book and some of the variations listed may be new to you. If so, it would make sense to experiment and get comfortable with these movements first before testing the ends of your strength; motor learning is a key aspect of this book with regard to getting the most from your training and not increasing the risk of injury.

Clearly, the caveat to these guidelines is that you do not have unlimited potential—you will hit what relates to your experience. However, I've found this data to be relatively accurate across the population I work with. It's also important to note that these goals assume that you have already built proper motor patterns with the squat, bench press, and deadlift—if you are not comfortable performing a one-rep max for maximal load, then these guidelines would be completely arbitrary and not aligned with your current level of experience.

In short, experienced lifters know that treating training as a marathon rather than a sprint is how we are able to both allow for consistent progression with metrics and stay mentally engaged in the process. Setting unreasonable goals sets the individual up to hit plateaus that can be a direct result of pushing too hard too often and adding a new level of stress to the nervous system.

BEST PRACTICES FOR GOAL SETTING

Setting goals and adhering to the training plan (or nutrition plan) that helps facilitate those goals is complex to say the least. One of the more critical pieces of the puzzle is mindset. Reframing one's mindset is often important, and although this is incredibly unique to the individual, I've seen some common mindset mistakes with the large majority of people who fail to hit their goals. According to the International Sports Sciences Association, these goal-setting actions are quite beneficial to anyone trying to reach new goals with their fitness:

- *Reframe the goal with a positive connotation.* Don't let yourself set goals like "not being weak" or "never eating junk food again." Success is more attainable with positive goals like getting stronger or eating more vegetables.
- *Don't be afraid to adjust goals as needed.* Making adjustments does not equate to not hitting your goal(s). This mindset is important to instill in yourself because not hitting a goal can cause loss of motivation. Always be prepared to make changes on the fly when needed.
- *Keep track of progress.* Write down tangible goals and monitor your progress toward them. Remember that all of your goals should

be measurable. When you're able to monitor your progress, your compliance and commitment to the goal will likely be much higher.

- *Do not punish failures.* Many people have the tendency to punish themselves when they fail to meet their goals, but this will only set you back further. Remove this idea, and be flexible—life is incredibly dynamic, and things happen.

- *Reward achievements.* We know that punishment is counter-productive, but having rewards for hitting goals is a great way to increase engagement. It's important and beneficial to celebrate small victories.

- *Do not focus on being perfect.* Perfection isn't realistic and results take time. Instead, continue to make incremental progress in your quest to reach your overall goals.

Adapted from International Sports Sciences Association, *Setting Fitness Goals is Essential to Long-Term Success* (Phoenix, AZ: ISSA).

In summary, creating realistic training goals may seem simple at first glance, but there are a number of "make-or-break" attributes to having things go smoothly. What's provided in this book is meant to reframe the goal setting process to set baseline expectations and metrics so you have a great place to start. It's important to remember that the crux of setting achievable goals is that they must be realistic. Before you go shooting for the stars (we've all been guilty of this), set goals you're almost certain you can hit within a four- to six-month time frame, hit those goals, reassess, and recalibrate new goals with a new date in sight. Although this may sound obvious, that couldn't be further from the truth. I've seen too many individuals fail to hit their goals after they got bogged down after missing their initial goals simply because they were not realistic.

PART II

THE EXERCISES

Chapter 5

Quad-Dominant Exercises

When we talk about quad-dominant exercises, the first one that usually comes to mind is the squat. However, in order to truly understand which muscle groups predominate during any given exercise, it's important to examine subtle nuances, such as the stance, that can change the reliance on agonist muscle groups. (In this case, a closer-stance squat would increase the degree of reliance on the quadriceps in comparison to a wider-stance squat, which would rely more on the hips and hamstrings.) Furthermore, these nuances should be considered in order to fully target specific areas; otherwise, a selected exercise may not be a truly quad-dominant choice.

With that said, even a movement like the front squat, which relies heavily on recruitment of the anterior chain, certainly includes contributions from posterior musculature such as the glutes and hamstrings. The front squat tends to be more quad-dominant than its back squat counterpart, but that's not to say that a back squat cannot be used strategically to target more quadriceps activation—it can. When it comes to exercise selection, subtle nuances such as foot position, stance, and position of the implement (in this case the barbell being situated anteriorly or posteriorly) can have a profound impact on the training effects.

In this chapter, we'll examine which exercises align with quadriceps development. This includes learning motor patterns with both bilateral and unilateral movements, improvements in maximal strength, and the ability to add lean tissue with hypertrophy schemes. Moreover, the exercises presented in this chapter are placed in chronological order, starting with unilateral variations and progressing to bilateral movements. Each included exercise is geared at targeting the quadriceps group, but other muscle groups will still have a role, acting as synergists or providing stability. (The split squat is a great example of an exercise that includes the quadriceps, the glutes, and to a lesser degree the hamstrings.) Additionally, the exercises progress in difficulty, starting from more basic variations (many of which you have likely seen or used before) to much more complex and difficult variations. If you have not mastered a unilateral movement like a split squat, progressing to a bilateral movement like a front squat wouldn't be prudent. I've included a lengthy list of quad-dominant exercises with additional exercise variations that can improve motor learning and prevent stagnation.

BACKWARD SLED DRAG

The backward sled drag is a great exercise that allows you to perform both strength and conditioning. This is accomplished by way of loco- motion, which elevates the heart rate to an aerobic level (around 60 to 70 percent of max heart rate for most people). Another important aspect of the sled drag is that it requires little skill to perform, making it a great fit for just about any level. If you're new to training and have access to a pulling sled, this is a great place to start. Moreover, even ad- vanced individuals can benefit from regular sled work to help facilitate recovery between higher-intensity sessions; because there is zero axial loading, this measure is easy to recover from.

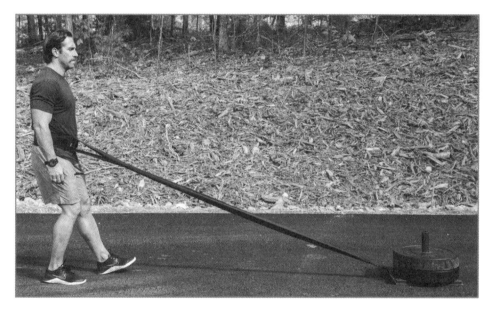

Instructions

- It is recommended to use a load (including the weight of the sled) of around 50 percent of your bodyweight. For example, a 200-pound (90 kg) person pulling a sled weighing the usual 25 pounds (11 kg) would add 75 additional pounds (34 kg) to the sled. However, you'll need to consider the surface you're pulling the sled on. If you're unable to move aggressively for all sets, you'll need to forgo these loading recommendations and instead use the heaviest load pos- sible while still being able to maintain consistency across all sets.
- Attach the sled straps to your weight belt and face the sled.
- Stand straight, initiating the movement using your arms and push- ing through the heels.

- Walk backward to pull the sled, pushing off with the heels on each rep to accentuate quadriceps activity (see figure).
- Use your arms as if you were running.

Protocol
Sets: 6
Reps: 30 yd (27 m)
Rest: 60-90 sec

Variation

Backward Sled Drag Backpedal

For the backward sled drag backpedal, follow the same mechanics as previously described, but as you get into the athletic stance, lower your position to a partial squat to add more quadriceps recruitment, which is advantageous for targeting the vastus medialis (the teardrop muscle of the quadriceps) (see figure). This variation is comparable to the position cornerbacks in American football spend a great deal of their time in on the field of play.

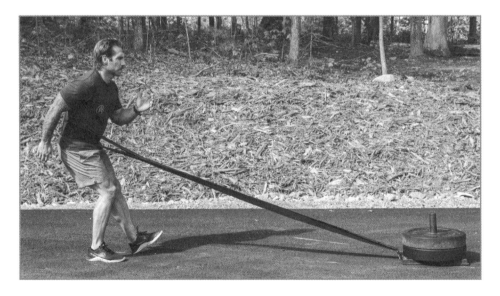

Protocol
Sets: 6
Reps: 30 yd (27 m)
Rest: 60-90 sec

DUMBBELL SPLIT SQUAT

No list of single-leg exercises is complete without a split squat, and the basic yet fundamental dumbbell split squat is important to learn and master. Even though dumbbell split squats are often considered remedial, they have a ton of value because they offer the ability to progress in terms of range of motion (ROM), loading capacity, and implements (dumbbells to barbells) so you can consistently make progressions when needed. Even the most basic exercise variation can offer a massive return on investment, and dumbbell split squats do not disappoint. Don't skip this exercise simply because the loading capacity is lower than using a barbell; these still have their place in proper program design for the lower body.

Instructions

- Stand holding a dumbbell in each hand.
- Step forward with one leg as you move into a 90/90 position, with the front upper leg close to parallel to the floor and the front shin vertical (see figure *a*).
- Lower yourself until your back knee hovers about 1 inch (2.5 cm) above the floor (see figure *b*).
- Push off with the front foot to return to the start position.
- Complete the repetitions on one leg; then switch sides.

Protocol

Sets: 3-4
Reps: 8-10
each side
Rest: 60 sec

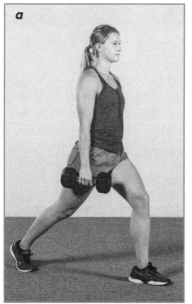
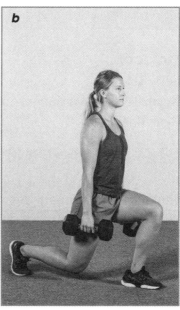

Variations

Front-Foot Elevated Split Squat

For more ROM, perform the front-foot elevated split squat by placing the front foot onto a riser of 2 to 4 inches (5 to 10 cm) and following the same mechanics as previously described (see figures *a* and *b*).

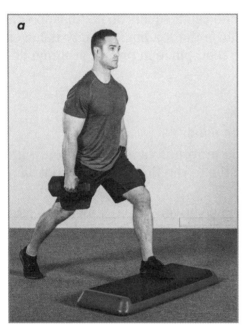
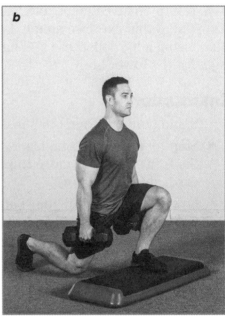

Protocol
Sets: 3-4
Reps: 8-12 each side
Rest: 60-90 sec

1-1/4 Dumbbell Split Squat

When performing the 1-1/4 dumbbell split squat, follow the same mechanics as previously described, but instead of returning to the start position, come up only a quarter of the way, lower yourself down again to the floor, and then come back up to the start position (see figures *a-d*). This constitutes 1 rep. The advantage of performing this variation is increased time under tension. Although its loading capacity is lower than that of the regular split squat, this variation can be used for higher-volume sets in more of a metabolic stress setting.

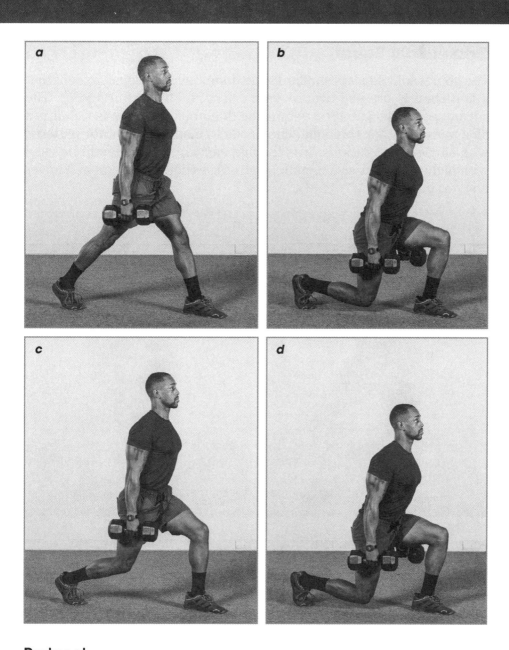

Protocol

Sets: 2-3

Reps: 12-15 each side (1 full ROM rep + 1/4 rep at the bottom of each rep = 1 rep)

Rest: 45-60 sec

Goblet Split Squat

The goblet split squat is similar to the dumbbell split squat, except that a kettlebell is pressed against your chest (see figures *a* and *b*). The advantage of this variation versus the dumbbell variation is that it is a nice regression for someone who needs to instill good motor patterns with single-leg variations (less loading capacity) but can still be used with higher-rep sets as a metabolic stress session at the end of a lower body training day.

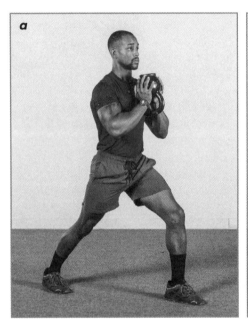
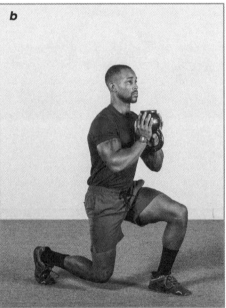

Protocol

Sets: 3-4
Reps: 10-15 each side
Rest: 45-60 sec

LANDMINE REVERSE LUNGE

Using a landmine offers the unique advantage of an anchor point that is farther away from you. The advantage of this is an increased level of loading capacity due to more stability being provided. Having the landmine appear early on in our single-leg quad-dominant exercise variations makes sense because of this increased stability. You can vary landmine single-leg exercises almost endlessly to create different challenges. In this case, repetitions are performed contralaterally, meaning you hold the barbell with one hand while the opposite leg performs the required work (e.g., you hold the sleeve of the barbell in your right hand while your left leg does the work).

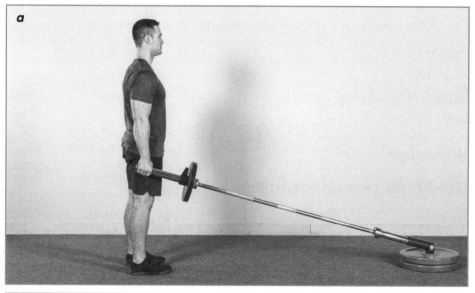

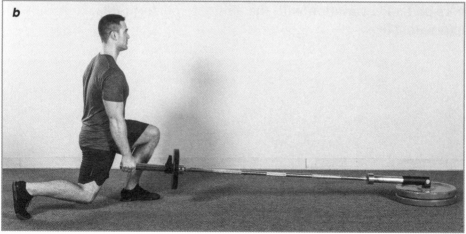

Instructions

- Stand facing the landmine, place one hand behind the collar of the barbell, and brace your abdominals (see figure *a*).
- Take a full step backward contralaterally (moving the leg opposite to the hand you're holding the barbell with) to a 90/90 lunge position (with the front shin vertical, just as in the split squat).
- Lower yourself until your back knee hovers about 1 inch (2.5 cm) above the floor (see figure *b*).
- Use the back leg to push yourself back to the start position.
- Keep your abdominals braced throughout the exercise.
- Complete the repetitions on one side; then switch legs.

Protocol
Sets: 3-4
Reps: 8-10 each side
Rest: 60 sec

Variation

Landmine Goblet Reverse Lunge

To perform the landmine goblet reverse lunge, follow the same mechanics as previously described, but hold the collar of the barbell with both hands in front of your chest (see figures *a* and *b*). You can alternate legs until all reps are complete. The benefit of holding the barbell against your chest is twofold: it creates more demand on the anterior core and adds variation with the ability to perform this exercise with alternating legs.

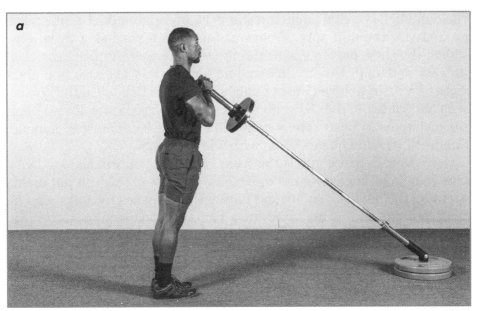

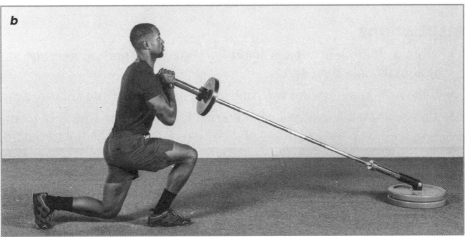

Protocol

Sets: 3-4
Reps: 8-10 each side
Rest: 60 sec

DUMBBELL WALKING LUNGE

The dumbbell walking lunge is a staple at any commercial gym, and as we increase the difficulty of our quad-dominant single-leg variations, adding dynamic movement to the lunge increases the need for both stability and skill. Due to its dynamic nature, this exercise will elicit higher levels of delayed onset muscle soreness (DOMS) in the quadriceps and glutes in the days after its use. This variation will also elicit a bigger spike in heart rate, which will increase local muscle demand. Dumbbell walking lunges come with a few caveats.

One caveat is that if you suffer from knee pain you will need to make sure your front knee does not move past your toes. This can put undue stress on the patellar tendon and flare up knee issues for folks who already present with generalized knee pain; the deceleration factor you have to contend with on each repetition can also make anterior knee over toe movement harder to avoid. Second, the back knee should not jam into the floor—each repetition should stop short of the back knee forcefully hitting the ground. While this is a good exercise, these caveats should be considered because no one exercise is the perfect fit for everyone.

Instructions

- Hold a dumbbell in each hand by your sides and brace your abdominals (see figure *a*).
- Take a big step forward with one leg, keeping your front shin vertical.
- Lower yourself until your back knee hovers about 1 inch (2.5 cm) over the floor (see figure *b*).

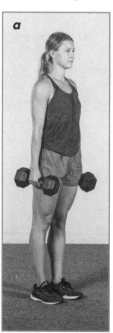
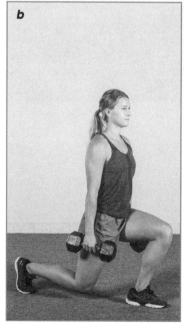

- Push off your back leg to bring that leg forward, and place that foot on the ground next to your front foot.
- Repeat the movement with the opposite leg, walking forward with each repetition.

Protocol

Sets: 3

Reps: 20 total steps (10 on each leg)

Rest: 60-90 sec

Variations

Walking Goblet Lunge

To perform the walking goblet lunge, follow the same mechanics as for the dumbbell walking lunge, but with a kettlebell pressed against your chest in a goblet position instead (see figures a and b). This variation is a nice regression for someone who needs to instill good motor patterns with single-leg variations (less loading capacity) but can also be used if higher-volume sets are the goal (metabolic stress setting), as has been discussed with previous single-leg variations.

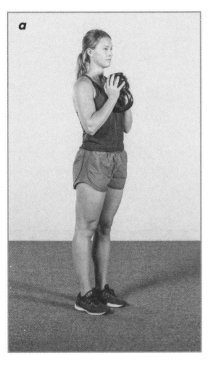
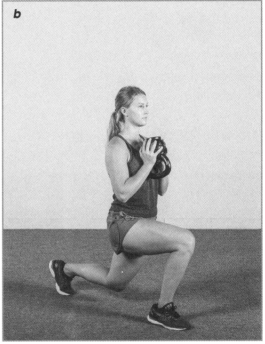

Protocol
Sets: 2-3
Reps: 20-30 total steps
Rest: 90 sec

Double Kettlebell Front Rack Walking Lunge

For a significantly higher demand on the anterior core, perform the walking lunge with two kettlebells in the front rack position (see figures *a* and *b*). Make sure your abdominals stay engaged the entire time. Keep in mind that this variation is an advanced single-leg progression that will challenge not only your anterior core but also your single-leg strength endurance with heavier loads.

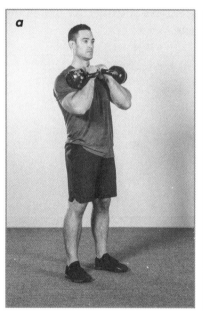
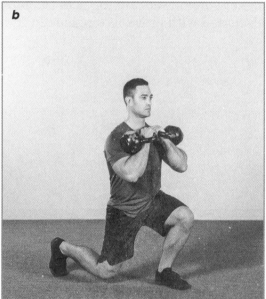

Protocol
Sets: 2-3
Reps: 20-30 total steps
Rest: 90 sec

The rear-foot elevated split squat, also known as the Bulgarian split squat, is a tough single-leg exercise to say the least and is a progression of the common split squat. While many associate "harder" exercises with progress, this typically isn't the case; more often it means that certain motor patterns must be dialed in first for safety and effectiveness. Much like dumbbell walking lunges, this exercise can be classified as quad-dominant, but the degree of stress placed on the glute complex is still high, so expect to experience high levels of DOMS in your glutes 48 to 72 hours after performing this exercise. This exercise is without a doubt the king of single-leg exercises and is often regarded as the be-all and end-all of single-leg strength. But again, what may be a great variation for one individual might be a mismatch for another.

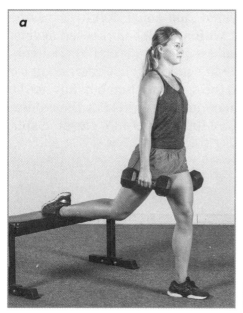
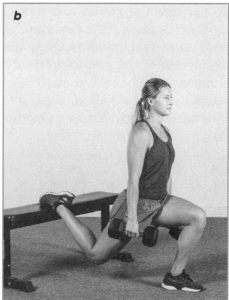

Instructions

- Stand facing away from a 16-inch (40 cm) bench, with a dumbbell in each hand.
- Step back with one leg to place the top of the foot on the bench (see figure *a*).
- Get into a 90/90 position where the front shin is vertical.
- Engage your anterior core by forcefully bracing your abdominals.
- Lower yourself until your back knee is 2 to 3 inches (5 to 8 cm) off the floor (see figure *b*). You may use a pad as a reference point if needed.

- With your back foot still on the bench, straighten your front leg to return to the start position.
- Complete the repetitions on one leg; then switch sides.

Protocol

Sets: 3-4
Reps: 6-10 each side
Rest: 90 sec

Variations

Goblet Rear-Foot Elevated Split Squat

To perform the goblet rear-foot elevated split squat, follow the same mechanics previously described, but with a kettlebell pressed against your chest in a goblet position instead (see figures *a* and *b*). The goblet version of the rear-foot elevated split squat is a nice regression for someone who has progressed beyond the split variation but may not be ready to use heavier loads in the form of dumbbells held by their sides. This variation can act as a teaching tool for the rear-foot elevated split squat.

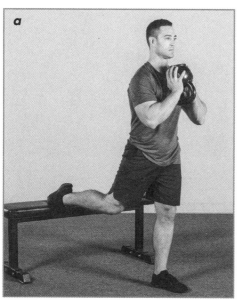 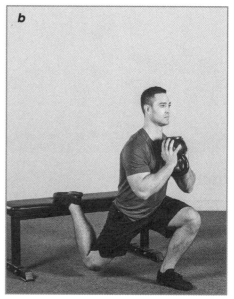

Protocol

Sets: 3-4
Reps: 8-10 each side
Rest: 60 sec

Barbell Front Rack Rear-Foot Elevated Split Squat

To perform the barbell front rack rear-foot elevated split squat, follow the same mechanics as previously described, but with a barbell in the front rack position (see figures *a* and *b*). The benefit of this variation is that using a barbell provides the opportunity to increase loading and lower body and anterior core demand.

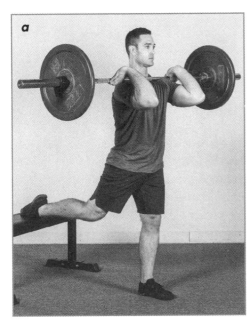
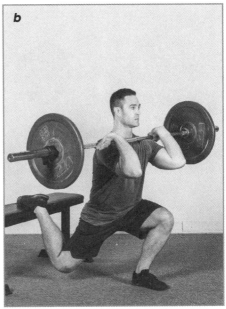

Protocol
Sets: 4-5
Reps: 6-8 each side
Rest: 90 sec to 2 min

As we advance up the single-leg training pyramid, any time we opt for using a barbell, loading capacity will be significantly higher. With increased ability to load your body comes higher demand systemically, as well as higher levels of requisite skill. (Higher loading capacity also brings higher levels of risk if you're not moving with great motor patterns to begin with.) Using a barbell in the back rack position to perform split squats increases loading capacity drastically because the load is farther away from your center of mass.

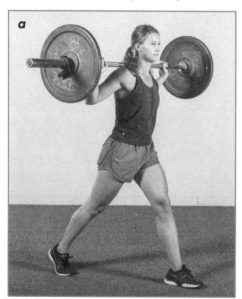 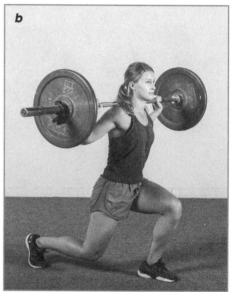

Instructions

- Stand with the barbell in the back rack position on your mid traps, and brace your abdominals. Your hands are roughly shoulder-width apart.
- Step back with one leg to move into a 90/90 position where the front shin is vertical (see figure *a*).
- Lower yourself until your back knee hovers about 1 inch (2.5 cm) above the floor (see figure *b*). You may use a pad as a reference point if needed.
- Push with your legs to return to the start position.
- Complete the repetitions on one leg; then switch sides.

Protocol

Sets: 5

Reps: 6-8 each side

Rest: 90 sec to 2 min

Variations

Front-Foot Elevated Barbell Back Rack Split Squat

For more ROM, perform a front-foot elevated barbell back rack split squat by placing a 2-inch (5 cm) riser under the front foot, and then follow the same mechanics as previously described (see figures *a* and *b*).

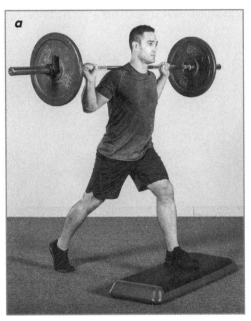
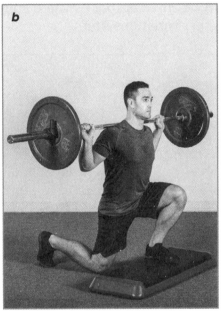

Protocol

Sets: 3-4

Reps: 8-10 each side

Rest: 60 sec

Rear-Foot Elevated Barbell Back Rack Split Squat

To perform the rear-foot elevated barbell back rack split squat, follow the same mechanics as previously described, but place the top of the back foot on a 16-inch (40 cm) bench behind you and lower yourself until your back knee is 2 to 3 inches (5 to 8 cm) off the floor (see figures *a* and *b*). This variation will give you the highest level of loading capacity of any rear-foot elevated split squat, so it's important to master all other variations first.

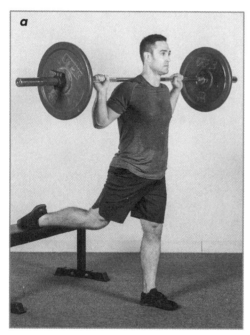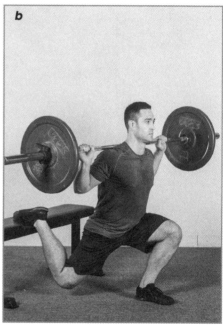

Protocol

Sets: 4-5

Reps: 6 each side

Rest: 90 sec to 2 min

BARBELL FRONT RACK REVERSE LUNGE

Now that we've talked about increasing loading capacity by way of using a barbell, adding a dynamic aspect to the lunge pattern is the next progression. The front rack reverse lunge is an incredible way to keep the knee from moving past the toes, so it's unlikely that they will exacerbate generalized knee pain in those who suffer from it. Moreover, barbell front rack reverse lunges offer a long list of benefits, such as better torso position (more upright) for more anterior core recruitment as well as recruitment of the rectus femoris, vastus lateralis, and vastus medialis—all critical to proper quadriceps development. Moreover, the dynamic nature of this movement makes it a great fit for athletes looking to improve performance.

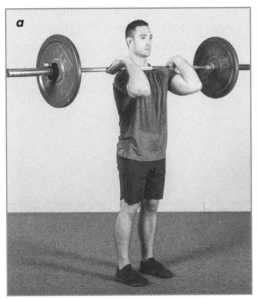 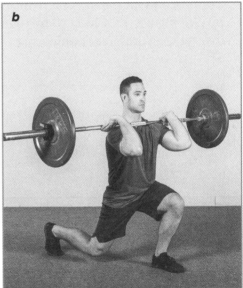

Instructions

- Stand with the barbell in the front rack position in front of your chest and brace your abdominals (see figure *a*). The hands are in a front rack position using a clean grip (double overhand, palms facing you) *or* the arms are crossed as in a bodybuilder front squat.
- Step back with one leg to move into a 90/90 position where the front shin is vertical.
- Lower yourself until your back knee hovers about 1 inch (2.5 cm) above the floor (see figure *b*). You may use a pad as a reference point if needed.

- Push with the legs to return to the start position.
- Complete repetitions on one leg; then switch sides.

Protocol
Sets: 5
Reps: 5 each side
Rest: 90 sec to 2 min

Variations

Front-Foot Elevated Front Rack Reverse Lunge

For more ROM, perform a front-foot elevated front rack reverse lunge by placing a 2- to 4-inch (5 to 10 cm) riser under both feet and then following the same mechanics as previously described (see figures *a* and *b*).

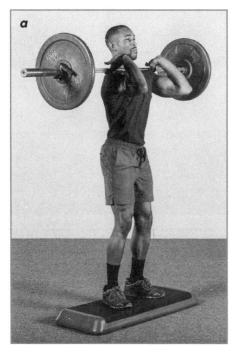
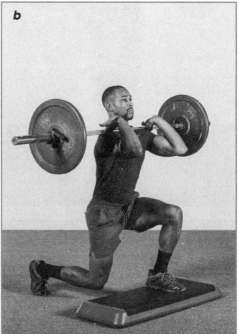

Protocol
Sets: 3-4
Reps: 8-10 each side
Rest: 90 sec

Zercher Barbell Reverse Lunge

To perform the Zercher barbell reverse lunge, place the barbell in the crook of your elbows, keeping the bar close to (touching) your abdominals, and then follow the same mechanics as for the barbell front rack reverse lunge (see figures *a* and *b*). The advantage of this exercise over other single-leg variations is the barbell placement, which increases demand on the upper back and anterior core. The Zercher variation is one that gets a lot of bad press because the barbell rests in the crook of the elbows, but it's an incredible variation for both single-leg patterns and the squat pattern.

Protocol

Sets: 4-5
Reps: 6-8 each side
Rest: 90 sec

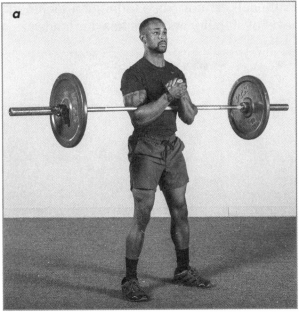

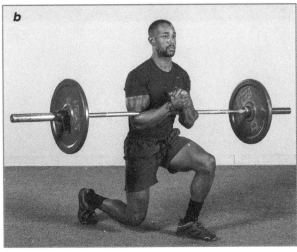

This exercise maintains constant tension on the adductors and quadriceps as all repetitions are performed in a squat position. This exercise is a frontal plane lateral squat that also focuses on the anterior core. Single-leg variations performed in the frontal plane are often low-hanging fruit for individuals since they are trained a fraction of the time compared to their sagittal plane counterparts. Although the benefits are comparable the execution and stress on inner thigh musculature is different.

This variation also is a great way to add variety in regard to single-leg frontal plane work but with higher loading capacity since you're using a landmine, which offers an added level of stability that a dumbbell or kettlebell cannot (the landmine attachment point equates to a higher level of stability and thus heavier loads are more likely).

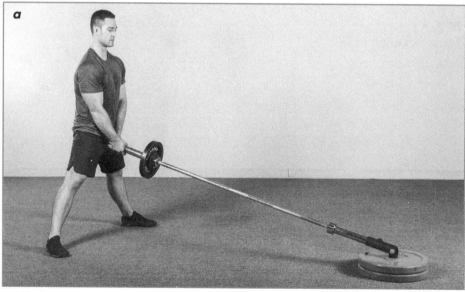

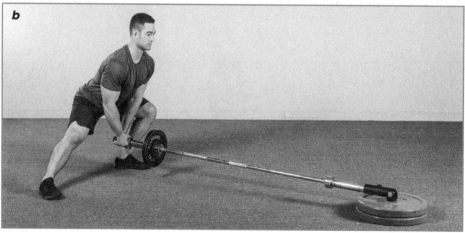

Instructions

- Hold the end of the barbell that is attached to a landmine between both legs. Assume an extra-wide sumo stance, keeping both feet flat on the floor (see figure *a*).
- Initiate the movement by pushing your hips back and driving your knee to the side the lunge is being performed (see figure *b*).
- Rotate left to right, maintaining the squat position as you move back and forth. This movement is performed in a low squat position throughout the entire exercise, meaning you do not return to fully standing between each rep.
- Both feet stay in contact with the floor at all times.

Protocol

Sets: 3-4
Reps: 6-8 each side
Rest: 90 sec

Variations

Goblet Lateral Squat

To perform the goblet lateral squat, hold a kettlebell pressed against your chest and follow the same mechanics as previously described, except you will return to the start position between each repetition (see figures *a* and *b*). Much like the landmine lateral squat there is constant tension on the adductors and quadriceps as all repetitions are performed in a squat position, but less so than that of the landmine variation since you'll be returning to a start position between each repetition.

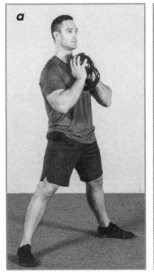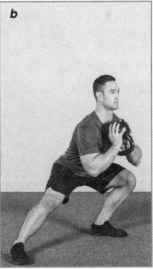

Protocol

Sets: 2-3
Reps: 8-10 each side
Rest: 90 sec

Landmine Goblet Lateral Squat

To perform the landmine goblet lateral squat, hold the landmine in a goblet position and press it against your chest, then follow the same mechanics as the landmine lateral squat (see figures *a* and *b*). This variation also gives you the added advantage of bar stability utilizing the landmine and thus higher loading capacity.

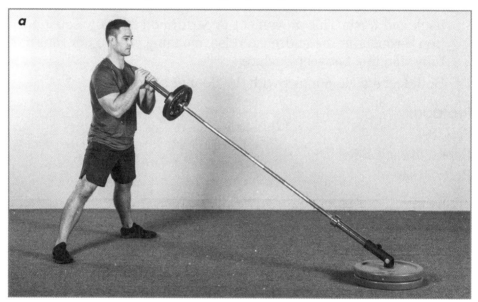

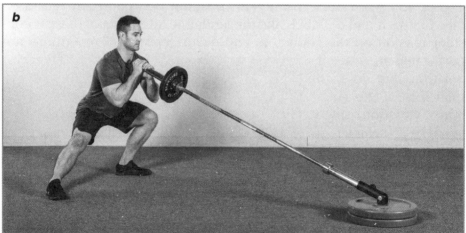

Protocol

Sets: 2-3
Reps: 8-10 each side
Rest: 90 sec

Now that we've covered staple unilateral movements that place a high degree of stress on the quadriceps group, the next step is to progress to bilateral movements such as the squat. However, instead of jumping right into a squat variation like front squats, we'll first look at effective ways to build the squat pattern. Enter goblet box squats. With a kettlebell or dumbbell pressed against your chest and the use of a box, you can build a great squat pattern before using higher-level variations. Goblet box squats do two things: (1) teach you to initiate your squat with a better lumbopelvic rhythm (i.e., pushing your hips back to the box) and (2) keep equal pressure in the forefoot and heels to ensure your squat pattern is not too quad-dominant.

Musculature dominance with squatting patterns is due in large part to your squat stance—a wider stance will elicit more recruitment of posterior musculature, such as the hamstrings, adductors, and glutes, whereas a closer stance will elicit more recruitment of anterior musculature such as the quadriceps. In this case, use whatever stance is most natural and comfortable for you. For many people, this is likely to be around shoulder-width apart. On the rare chance that you're more comfortable with a wide stance, I'd encourage you to play with a closer stance if quadriceps development is your goal. Additionally, goblet box squats require you to push your hips back to the box, pause slightly on the box, and then stand up. To be clear, this is not a "touch and go" squat variation where you simply tap the box and then go through concentric ROM.

Instructions

- Stand with your feet shoulder-width apart and face away from a 14- to 16-inch (35 to 40 cm) box or bench. Stand roughly 3 to 4 inches (8 to 10 cm) from the box (see figure *a*).

- Hold a dumbbell or kettlebell against your chest with both hands (goblet position).

- Bend your knees and lower yourself, push-

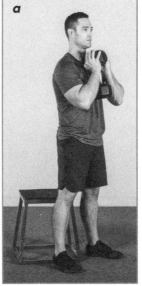
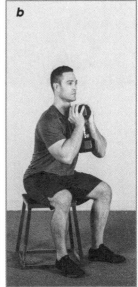

ing your hips back toward the box while maintaining a vertical torso.

- The ideal squat depth is parallel or below, but the depth you choose should not impair your ability to maintain a neutral spine.
- The shins should remain somewhat vertical; the box will allow you to ensure this as your hips and hamstrings are actively engaged to a higher degree than the goblet squat without a box variation.
- Pause for 1 to 2 seconds, with your backside touching the box, while keeping your back tight and core engaged—there should be an arch in your lower back; at no point should your lumbar spine round over (see figure *b*).
- Return to the start position by pushing down through your heels and straightening your legs.

Protocol
Sets: 3-4
Reps: 10-12
Rest: 60 sec

Variations

Goblet Squat

To perform the goblet squat, hold a kettlebell in the goblet position against your chest with feet roughly shoulder-width apart and toes

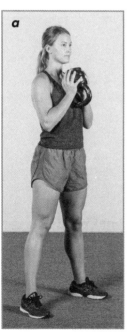
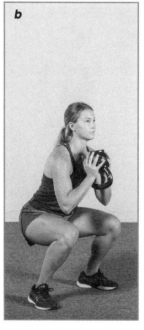

slightly pointed out (see figure *a*). Initiate the movement by pushing your hips back and going through a full ROM that allows for maximum ROM based on your individual anthropometrics (the maximum depth you can achieve while still maintaining a neutral spine) (see figure *b*). The goblet squat is not only a great teaching tool to learn the squat pattern but a great tool for hypertrophy of the lower body.

Protocol

Sets: 3-4

Reps: 12-15

Rest: 60 sec

Double Kettlebell Box Squat

To engage the anterior core to a higher degree, perform the goblet box squat with two kettlebells in the front rack position and the elbows in close proximity to the abdominals (see figures *a* and *b*). Make sure your abdominals stay engaged the entire time.

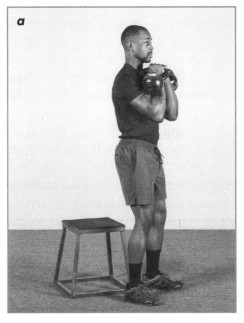 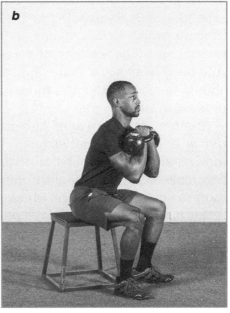

Protocol

Sets: 3-4

Reps: 8-10

Rest: 90 sec

ANDERSON FRONT SQUAT

The Anderson front squat uses pins in a squat rack to allow you to start from the bottom position of your squat or at your sticking point, which varies for each person, and then stand. Anderson front squat variations offer a number of great benefits that differ from those of the traditional front squat, which consists of both a lowering and a lifting phase. The movements of the Anderson front squat are more concentric based.

Anderson front squats are a great way to build absolute strength, which is an integral part of well-rounded maximal strength. Moreover, concentric movements like Anderson front squats allow you to use different heights, different bars, and accommodating resistance (bands, chains, or both at the same time). You'll notice that you'll also be able to work up to supramaximal loads (loads that go beyond your one-repetition max) depending on the starting height of the movement and to work partial ROM movements to facilitate high levels of motor-unit recruitment. The strategy of using movements like the supramaximal Anderson front squat that emphasize the concentric phase of the squat should be used with care, though, because it's very demanding on the nervous system.

Another great benefit of Anderson front squats is that they are effective at building lockout strength because you specifically target your individual sticking points and vary the joint angles that may be less favorable based on your anthropometrics. For example, it's not uncommon to see individuals get stuck finishing the top half of their squat. If this is the case for you, I encourage you to work in this ROM to improve these limitations.

Anderson front squats also allow you to learn how to develop tension. Maximal effort work requires the ability to create tension, and oftentimes this aspect of training gets forgotten. Concentric movements force you to develop tension prior to initiating your movement because you start from a disadvantage, unable to use the stretch reflex.

Lastly, because you omit the eccentric phase, Anderson front squats do not cause the same amount of muscular soreness; this will improve your ability to recover between training sessions.

Instructions

- Set the squat rack pins at your desired height. You will need to test and experiment with this prior to adding any load to the barbell. If you're new to Anderson front squat variations, position the barbell so that you start with a parallel squat—hip crease parallel to your knees.

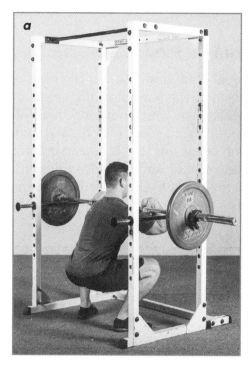 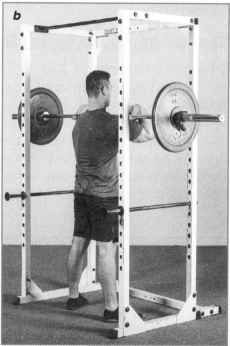

- Position yourself under the barbell, using a front rack position (clean grip or arms crossed—whichever is most comfortable), and brace your anterior core (see figure *a*).
- Initiate leg drive while keeping pressure in your heels and stand up (see figure *b*). Resist the tendency to lean forward or shift weight to your toes.
- Once you're fully standing, lower the weight back to the pins, or, if performing a 1-repetition set, simply rack the barbell.

Protocol

Sets: Build in weight over the course of 5 sets
Reps: 5RM
Rest: 2.5 min

Variation

Zercher Anderson Squat From Low Pins

To perform the Zercher Anderson squat from low pins, set the pins as for the Anderson front squat, but position the barbell in the crook of your elbows with the barbell pressed against your body, and then follow the same mechanics as the Anderson front squat (see figures *a-c*). The benefits of the Zercher Anderson squat are that it places greater demand on the upper back and anterior core and provides you with variability because you can start the movement from different positions (the height of the pins can be varied).

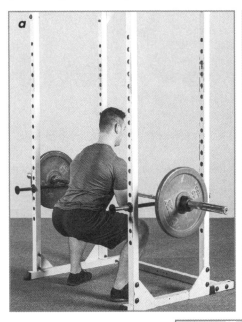
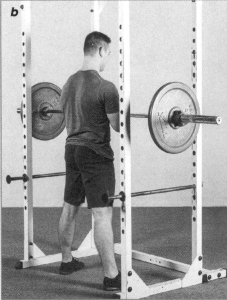
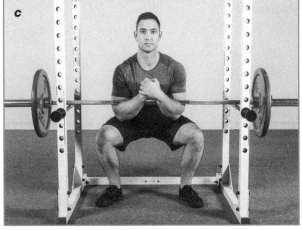

Protocol
Sets: 9
Reps: Build to a 1RM
Rest: 2-3 min

The barbell front box squat is the king of bilateral quad-dominant exercises, in my humble opinion. First, box squats offer a number of great benefits, such as breaking up the eccentric and concentric phases of the lift; the ability to build to your starting strength since you are not employing the elastic abilities of the stretch-shortening cycle; and the ability to decrease loading capacity, which can prevent articular wear and tear. These variations use your natural squat stance (not a wide stance) to a parallel or slightly below parallel box (14 to 16 inches [35 to 40 cm] in most cases).

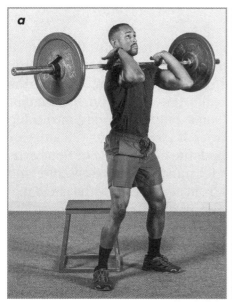 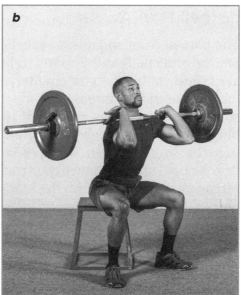

Instructions

- Stand with your feet shoulder-width apart, facing away from a 14- to 16-inch (35 to 40 cm) box or bench (see figure *a*). Stand roughly 3 to 4 inches (8 to 10 cm) from the box.
- Hold the barbell in the front rack position, either with a clean grip or with arms crossed, holding the barbell in place.
- While maintaining a vertical torso, bend your knees and lower yourself, pushing your hips back toward the box.
- The ideal squat depth is parallel or below, but the depth you choose should not impair your ability to maintain a neutral spine, and your shins should be somewhat vertical throughout the lowering phase.
- Pause for 1 to 2 seconds, with your backside touching the box, while keeping your back tight and core engaged (see figure *b*). There should be a slight arch in your lower back—at no point should your lumbar spine round over.

- Return to the start position by pushing down through your heels and straightening your legs.

Protocol

Sets: 5-8
Reps: 1-5RM
Rest: 2.5 min

Variations

Barbell Front Squat

The barbell front squat is an excellent teaching tool to train the squat pattern and one that I've found to be more practical for most individuals versus its back squat counterpart. The reason being, loading the barbell anteriorly versus posteriorly puts less stress on the lumbar spine, so there is less chance of the squat pattern turning into a hip hinge (torso excessively leaning forward). It also stresses the anterior core to a higher degree. With this is mind, the application of this variation for both strength and hypertrophy for most individuals is safer and more effective. To perform the barbell front squat, follow the same mechanics as previously described for the barbell front box squat but focus on mechanics (see figures *a* and *b*). The depth you choose should not impair your ability to maintain a neutral spine, and your shins should be somewhat vertical throughout the lowering phase.

Protocol

Sets: Build in weight over the course of 5-8 sets
Reps: 1-5RM
Rest: 2-3 min

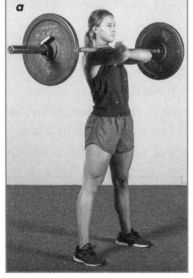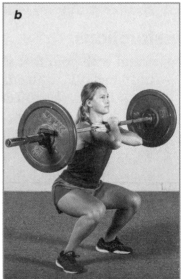

Barbell Front Box Squat Clusters

To perform a barbell front box squat cluster set, you'll perform the prescribed repetitions (in this case 3, 2, and 1), then rerack the weight and rest a predetermined amount of time between cluster sets. For example, unrack the weight, perform 3 front box squats, rerack the weight, wait 15 seconds, unrack the weight, perform 2 repetitions, rerack the weight, wait 15 seconds. Finally, unrack the weight, perform 1 repetition, rerack the weight, then rest until fully recovered (approximately 3 minutes). This will allow you to perform higher volumes of work with less chance of incurring mechanical breakdown.

Protocol
Sets: 3
Reps: 3.2.1 (15 sec) @ 80%-85% of 1RM
Rest: 3 min

1-1/4 FRONT SQUAT

Last but not least, the 1-1/4 front squat provides all the benefits of the anterior-loaded front squat plus the additional time under tension on each repetition from performing an extra quarter squat. Adding the quarter squat effectively reduces loading capacity, which to some may sound counterintuitive, but the reality is that at times decreasing loading capacity improves trainability of movement due to shorter recovery between sessions with a reduced cost on both the muscular system and the central nervous system. Because time under tension is higher with this variation, you may find it prudent to go with the arms-crossed front rack position if you lack upper body mobility. Lastly, this varia-

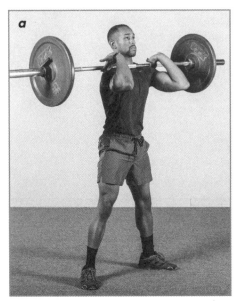

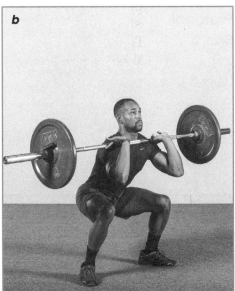

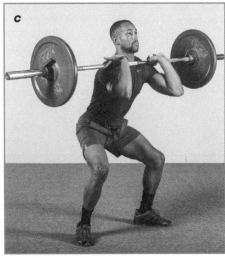

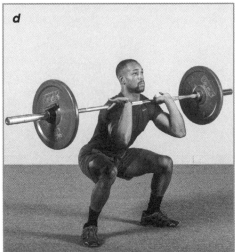

tion is incredibly demanding on the quadriceps, in particular the vastus medialis. This exercise is optimally performed with a closer-than-normal squat stance.

Instructions

- Stand with your feet shoulder-width apart or narrower (see figure *a*).
- Hold the barbell in the front rack position. This can be performed using a clean grip or with arms crossed if your front rack mobility is limited, holding the barbell in place.
- While keeping your torso vertical, bend your knees and lower yourself by pushing your hips back, keeping your back tight and core engaged. There should be a slight arch in your lower back—at no point should your lumbar spine round over.
- The ideal squat depth is parallel or below, but the depth you choose should not impair your ability to maintain a neutral spine (see figure *b*).
- Come up only a quarter of the way rather than returning to the start position (see figure *c*).
- Lower yourself down again (see figure *d*), pause for 1 to 2 seconds, and then come back up to the start position by pushing down through your heels and straightening your legs.

Protocol

Sets: 5
Reps: 4RM (1 full ROM rep + 1/4 rep at the bottom of each rep = 1 rep)
Rest: 2.5 min

Variation

1-1/4 Front Box Squat

To perform the 1-1/4 front box squat, start by standing facing away from a 14- to 16-inch (35 to 40 cm) box or bench and stand roughly 3 to 4 inches (8 to 10 cm) from the box (see figure *a*). Follow the same mechanics as the 1-1/4 front squat, except when you lower, pause for 1 to 2 seconds with your backside touching the box (see figure *b*). Then, keeping pressure in your heels, stand up a quarter of the distance to standing to perform a quarter squat (see figure *c*), then lower back down to the box (see figure *d*). Pause, then return to the start position. This constitutes 1 rep. The benefits of this variation are twofold: it increases time under tension for greater hypertrophy of the quadriceps, and it is a great way to build rigidity in the bottom of your squat.

Protocol

Sets: 6

Reps: Build to a heavy set of 3 (1 full ROM rep + 1/4 rep at the bottom of each rep = 1 rep)

Rest: 2-3 min

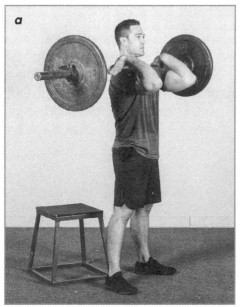

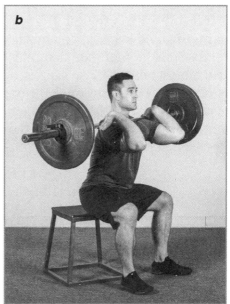

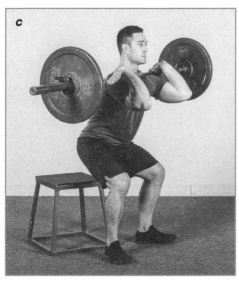

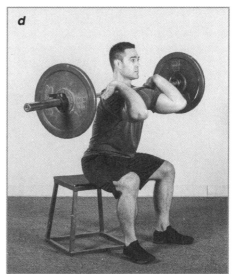

In conclusion, this list of quad-dominant exercises can serve a multitude of functions within your program design, such as creating balance within a training plan, providing novelty of variations to keep the training engaging, and keeping you moving forward with both progressions and regressions in your exercise selection. The final caveat to remember is that almost none of these exercises are 100 percent quad-dominant. There is certainly contribution from opposing muscle groups—the rear-foot elevated split squat is a great example—but knowing that the quadriceps will certainly predominate in most of these exercises is important for designing effective training plans.

Chapter 6

Hip-Dominant Exercises

As we have said before, individuals with a higher number of muscular imbalances generally find it advantageous to prioritize training hip-dominant exercises; however, no two individuals are exactly the same, so this may not be true for everyone. In addition to lowering the incidence of lower back pain, training the posterior chain muscles has definitive benefits such as improving posture and strength and bringing people into more extension-based positions to help remediate against the countless number of hours people are sitting on a daily basis. Although posterior chain training is clearly important, that does not mean you should totally disregard training the anterior portions of your lower body; otherwise you might be leaving results on the table.

Anecdotally, a 2:1 posterior versus anterior training of the lower body has been a ratio I've witnessed being accurate across a wide range of the population. In the past decade and even longer, the large majority of the clients I've come across came from traditional endurance backgrounds running the occasional 5K or 10K or simply using jogging as their main mode of exercise. With this prior knowledge, pinpointing where these individuals tend to present weaknesses and structural imbalances is relatively straightforward. An easy assessment is to examine your motor patterns and movement deficiencies with a simple hip hinge test. People with endurance backgrounds will typically present more knee dominance, meaning they rely more on their anterior chain and initiate movement by pushing their knees forward. Someone who has a background playing high-level American football tends to be more hip-dominant, presenting with a better ability to engage posterior musculature such as the hamstrings and glutes. While this is not always the case, the specificity of one's sport (endurance sports or American football in this case) often helps give an indication of where to start in terms of musculature deficiencies. These are key factors when trying to understand where someone should devote more of their training. An equal distribution of squatting and hinging patterns is a safe bet, but if all else fails, increase the volume of hip hinge dominant patterns. In many situations, by simply adding more volume to hip-dominant movements, lower back issues start to clear up and improvements can be seen in squat and deadlift patterns.

The exercise choices provided in this chapter are both unilateral (single-leg patterns) and bilateral (multijoint patterns), in addition to some hybrid-style movements (for example, sled pulls are in essence unilaterally demanding but also add the element of conditioning with benefits to the aerobic system). While it may not seem straightforward now on how to plug these exercises into your programming, this will become clear once you see the actual programs in part III. Furthermore, the exercises in this chapter are variations to many staple hip-dominant movements. For example, the Romanian deadlift (RDL) is a staple hip hinge pattern variation found in many great exercise programs; however, variations to the RDL, such as an RDL with a different foot stance or the use of accommodating resistance, are less common. The latter will be presented in this book, although that is not to say that the root variation is not equally as important.

FORWARD SLED DRAG

The forward sled drag is an exercise that emphasizes the musculature of the hips, hamstrings, calves, and quadriceps, with the majority of the forward leg drive powered by the glutes and hamstrings. This exercise is an incredible way to train this musculature without eccentric loading and high amounts of tissue breakdown; it can therefore have a massive carryover to bilateral movements like squats and deadlifts with very low risk of overtraining. Much like backward sled drags, which we learned about in the previous chapter, forward sled drags are low-skill and beneficial at all training levels. Forward sled drag variations deliver more stress on the hamstrings, glutes, and spinal erectors and can be used in multiple scenarios, such as strength, conditioning, and recovery-based sessions. They are easy to recover from, making them a great fit to help athletes maintain high levels of strength and aerobic fitness within their season of play.

This exercise can have a wide variety of applications in program design. There aren't many tasks the sled couldn't be useful for. For strength purposes, for instance, heavier loading with shorter distances can be implemented (6 to 10 sets × 40 to 60 yards [37 to 55 m]). Conversely, for strength endurance, the sled can be used for longer distances (3 to 4 sets × 100 to 200 yards [90 to 180 m]), and if recovery is the goal or the sled isn't being used to bridge the gap between training sessions, distances of up to 1 mile (1.6 km) with light loads can be used.

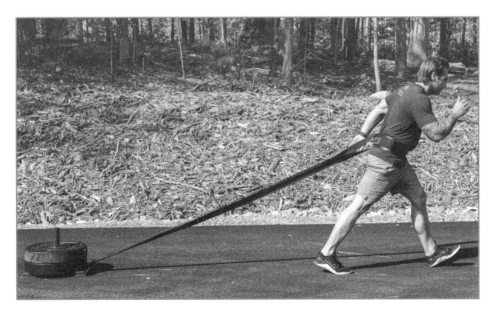

Instructions

- Attach the sled straps to a weight belt and face away from the sled. This ensures the glutes and hamstrings will predominate in the movement.
- Walk or sprint forward, using a powerful leg drive with a heel-to-toe action (see figure).
- Use your arms as if you're sprinting; arms are positioned at 90 degrees.

Protocol

Sets: 6-10
Reps: 60 yd (55 m)
Rest: 60-90 sec

Variations

Forward Sled Drag for Strength

To perform the forward sled drag for strength, follow the same mechanics as described previously, but the amount of load will change. For strength work, use three-quarters of your bodyweight, including the weight of the sled. The common pulling sled weighs 25 pounds (11 kg), so a 200-pound (90 kg) person would use 125 additional pounds (57 kg) on the sled. However, you'll need to consider the surface you're pulling the sled on. If you're unable to move aggressively for all sets, you'll need to forgo these loading recommendations and instead use the heaviest load possible while still being able to maintain consistency across all sets.

Protocol

Sets: 6
Reps: 60 yd (55 m)
Rest: 60 sec

Forward Sled Drag for Strength Endurance

To perform the forward sled drag for strength endurance, follow the same mechanics as described previously, but the amount of load will change. For strength endurance, use 25 to 50 percent of your body-weight, including the weight of the sled. The common pulling sled weighs 25 pounds (11 kg), so a 200-pound (90 kg) person would use 25 to 75 additional pounds (11 to 34 kg) on the sled. However, you'll need to consider the surface you're pulling the sled on. If you're unable to move aggressively for all sets, you'll need to forgo these loading recommendations and instead use the heaviest load possible while still being able to maintain consistency across all sets.

Protocol
Sets: 3-4
Reps: 200 yd (180 m)
Rest: 60-90 sec

Forward Sled Drag for Aerobic Conditioning

To perform the forward sled drag for aerobic conditioning, follow the same mechanics as described previously, but the amount of load will change. For aerobic conditioning, use 10 to 25 percent of your body-weight, including the weight of the sled. The common pulling sled weighs 25 pounds (11 kg), so a 200-pound (90 kg) person would use an empty sled or 25 pounds (11 kg) on the sled. However, you'll need to consider the surface you're pulling the sled on. If you're unable to move aggressively for all sets, you'll need to forgo these loading recommendations and instead use the heaviest load possible while still being able to maintain consistency across all sets.

Protocol
Sets: As few as possible
Reps: 1 mile (1.6 km) total for time
Rest: As needed

The classic cable pull-through allows you to ingrain proper hip hinge motor patterns while training the musculature of the glutes and hamstrings. The cable pull-through is a simple way for you to learn how to properly hip hinge with less risk of injury than an exercise like a deadlift, which presents the same pattern with higher degrees of loading and musculature. In this case, we break down the hip hinge pattern into a more simplistic form using a cable attached to a machine behind you. This exercise isn't new for most people, but it works well in higher-repetition scenarios because the glutes respond well to higher volume due to higher concentrations of slow-twitch muscle fibers. Aim for repetitions of 15 to 20 per set. Another benefit of this exercise is that it does *not* require the use of a cable machine; a variation can be done at home by simply affixing a moderate to heavy band to a fixed location.

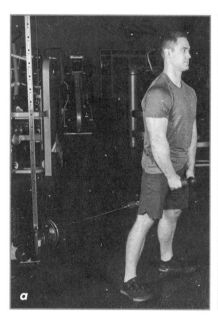
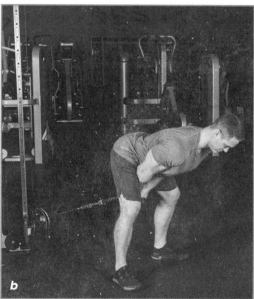

Instructions

- Stand with your feet slightly farther than shoulder-width apart, facing away from the cable machine with the cable between your legs.
- Grasp the cable with both hands, and walk forward until there is tension and no slack in the cable (see figure *a*).
- Hinge at the hips and bend your knees slightly as you allow your hands to move back behind you (see figure *b*). Think of sitting back, not down. Your hips lead the movement, not your knees; the knees stay unlocked but static.

- Arch your lower back and tuck your chin.
- Once you feel a stretch in your hamstrings to indicate you're at the end of your range of motion (ROM), reverse the movement by squeezing your glutes to return to standing.

Protocol

Sets: 3-4

Reps: 15-20

Rest: 60 sec

Variation

Banded Pull-Through

To perform the banded pull-through, follow the same mechanics as described previously, but step forward to create tension on the band. There should be constant tension through full ROM, so you'll need to step forward far enough that there is tension as you hip hinge as well as at your start position when you are standing up straight (see figures *a* and *b*).

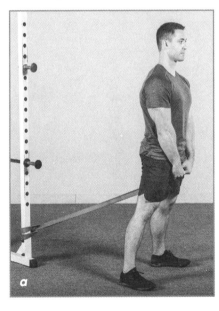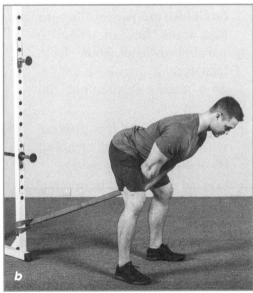

Protocol

Sets: 4

Reps: 25

Rest: 45-60 sec

The single-leg glute hip thrust is a great exercise to target and isolate the glutes. With many hip-dominant exercises, it's nearly impossible to isolate one muscle group, and for many people, the hamstrings will predominate over the glutes. When working unilaterally, the likelihood of isolating the glutes becomes more realistic, and there is less chance that lack of movement proficiency will be a limiting factor. Enter the single-leg glute hip thrust off a bench—an excellent way to isolate and train the glutes unilaterally with less chance of the hamstrings overpowering the glutes. Like the pull-through variations, glute hip thrusts work best when programmed with higher repetitions, typically in the 10+ range.

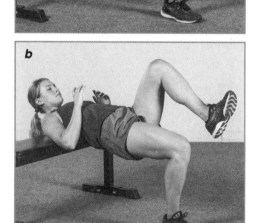

Instructions

- Sit on the floor in front of the long side of a standard-height weight bench.
- Raise your body to place your mid back fully on the bench. Place your feet about hip-width apart, and lift your hips until they are close to parallel to the floor. Both legs remain at about 90-degree angles throughout the movement.
- Lift one leg off the ground, with the knee bent at about 90 degrees (see figure *a*).
- Lower your hips until your backside is a few inches above the floor.
- Initiate an upward motion by thrusting the hip of the working leg upward, tucking your chin and squeezing your glute at the top (see figure *b*).
- Complete the repetitions on one side; then switch legs.

Protocol
Sets: 2-3
Reps: 12-15 each side
Rest: 60 sec

Variation

1-1/2 Single-Leg Glute Hip Thrust

When performing the 1-1/2 single-leg glute hip thrust, follow the same mechanics as previously described, but instead of returning directly to the start position, first come up only half of the way, lower yourself down again to the bottom position, and then return to the start position (see figures *a-d*). This constitutes 1 rep.

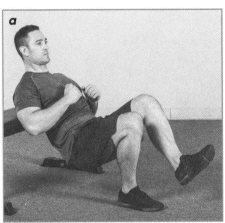
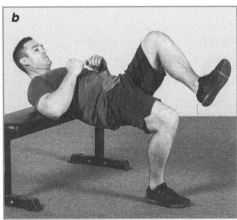
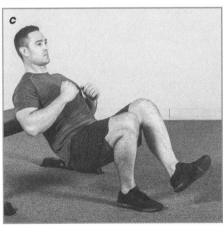
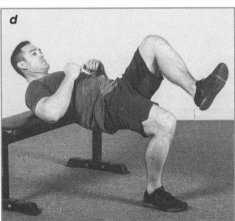

Protocol

Sets: 3-4

Reps: 8-10 each side (1 full ROM rep + 1/2 rep at the bottom of each rep = 1 rep)

Rest: 60 sec

The barbell glute hip thrust is a bilateral exercise that targets the hamstrings and to a higher degree the glute complex. Like the single-leg glute hip thrust, this exercise is effective because of its ability to isolate and target the glutes. Barbell glute hip thrusts have made quite a name for themselves thanks to people like Dr. Bret Contreras, a strength coach and author who gained popularity from this exercise and his work to bring direct glute training to the forefront of strength training. Barbell glute hip thrusts utilize all four actions of the glutes—hip external rotation, hip abduction, hip extension, and posterior pelvic tilt. There are a few pointers for reaping the benefits of this exercise. First, use a bench or a box with a height of 12 to 16 inches (30 to 40 cm). Second, don't sacrifice ROM for load—it's common to see people miss-ing 10 to 15 percent of end ROM just to use heavier load-ing. Additionally, although this variation could be programmed for heavier work (3- to 6-rep max), I've found this variation to be more effective in the 8- to 12-rep range and have gone as high as 20-rep sets, so feel free to experiment.

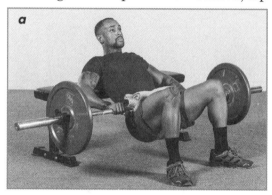

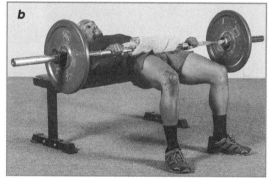

Instructions

- Sit on the floor in front of the long side of a standard-height weight bench.
- Raise your body to place your mid back fully on the bench and your feet about hip-width apart. The legs should be at about 90-degree angles throughout the entire movement.
- Place a standard barbell with a pad or folded towel over your pelvis (see figure *a*).
- Push through the heels and use the glutes to thrust the hips upward until they are parallel to the floor (see figure *b*).
- Tuck your chin and squeeze your glutes at the top.
- Lower your hips until your backside is about 1 to 2 inches (2.5 to 5 cm) above the floor. That's 1 rep.

Protocol

Sets: 4-5

Reps: 8-10

Rest: 90 sec

Variation

1-1/4 Barbell Glute Hip Thrust

When performing the 1-1/4 barbell glute hip thrust, follow the same mechanics as previously described, but instead of returning to the start position, come up only a quarter of the way, lower yourself down again to the floor, and then back up to the start position (see figures *a-d*). This constitutes 1 rep.

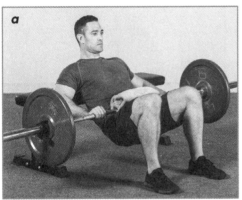
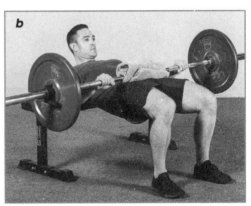
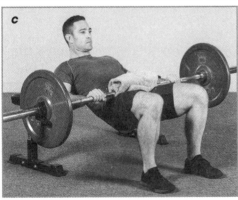
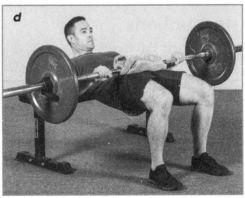

Protocol

Sets: 3-4

Reps: 10-12 (1 full ROM rep + 1/4 rep at the top of each rep = 1 rep)

Rest: 90 sec

The 45-degree back raise is a great exercise to isolate the glutes with less chance of technical error. The 45-degree back extension machine is a common piece of equipment found at any commercial gym. The back raise has been shown via electromyography readings to elicit massive amounts of gluteus maximus activation (Contreras 2019), making it a clear choice to improve hip extension and glute development. It also offers many variations without much additional equipment.

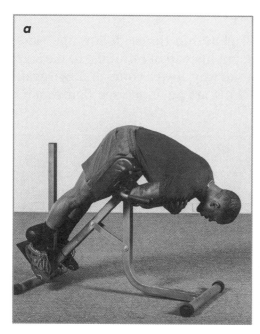
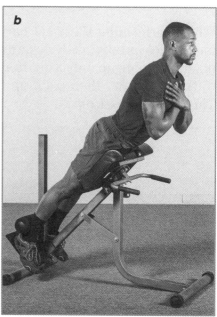

Instructions

- Adjust the machine so that the tops of your thighs rest against the pad, and place your feet in front of the ankle pad. Stand tall and brace your core.
- With your arms crossed across your chest, hinge at the hips to lower your upper body toward the floor until you feel a slight stretch in your hamstrings (see figure a). Keep your back straight.
- Raise yourself, keeping your chin tucked and back straight (see figure b).
- Squeeze your glutes at the top of the movement.

Protocol

Sets: 3-4
Reps: 12-15
Rest: 60 sec

Variations

Medicine Ball Loaded Back Raise

To perform the medicine ball loaded back raise, follow the same mechanics as previously described, but hold a medicine ball at your chest throughout the exercise (see figures *a* and *b*).

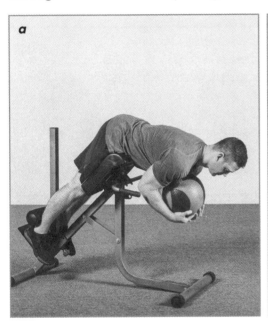
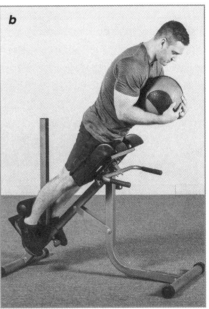

Protocol

Sets: 4

Reps: 15-20

Rest: 60 sec

Single-Leg Back Raise

The single-leg back raise is executed with one leg rather than two. To perform this exercise, set up in a 45-degree back extension machine with one leg behind the back plate and the opposite leg on top of the back plate. This movement is executed in the same fashion with one leg as opposed to both legs being locked into place (see figures *a* and *b*).

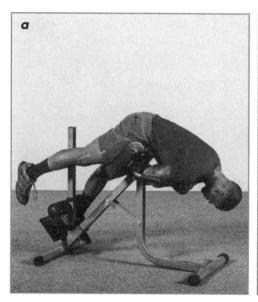
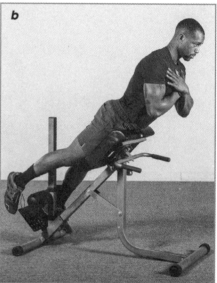

Protocol

Sets: 4

Reps: 8-10 each side

Rest: 60 sec

The Romanian deadlift is a staple movement for hammering the hamstrings for just about any experienced lifter, but its single-leg counterpart is less known. The single-leg version is an important variation to train the hamstrings and the hip hinge pattern in a contralateral fashion (with the working leg and arm holding the barbell opposing). Because learning to move unilaterally is important to ensure symmetry and balance before attempting heavier bilateral movements, this variation is listed before the standard Romanian deadlift. As we mentioned in chapter 5, the landmine offers you the ability to train with an anchor point that's farther away, which creates a higher level of stability and therefore an increase in loading capacity. With single-leg variations, less stability is often necessary to improve symmetry, but variations like the single-leg landmine Romanian deadlift are great for changing loading capacity and trainability. Less stability is *not* always the answer when it comes to improving single-leg strength, making this a viable option to train the hamstrings and the hip hinge pattern.

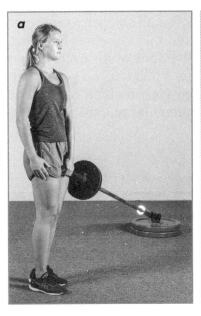 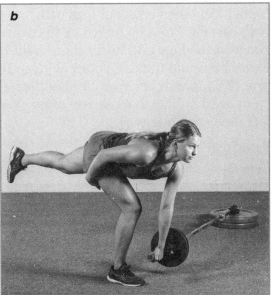

Instructions
- Stand with your side facing the end of the barbell that is opposite the landmine attachment.
- Grasp and lift the barbell with the hand closest to it (see figure *a*).
- Hinge at the hips and lower the weight to the floor while lifting the leg closest to the barbell off the floor behind you so that you're working only the far leg (see figure *b*).

- Arch your lower back and tuck your chin. The working leg is unlocked but static; all movement comes from the hips, not the knees.
- When you get to your end ROM, hinge back up to standing while lowering the back leg. Keep your body in a long line from head to back heel as you move.
- Complete the repetitions on one leg; then switch legs.

Protocol

Sets: 3-4
Reps: 8-10 each side
Rest: 60 sec

Variation

Split Stance Landmine Romanian Deadlift

To perform the split stance landmine Romanian deadlift, stand with the barbell held between your legs with two hands and stagger your stance with one leg 3 to 4 inches (8 to 10 cm) behind the other (see figure *a*). Hinge at the hips and lower the weight to the floor while arching your lower back and tucking your chin (see figure *b*). When you get to your end ROM, hinge back up to standing. Keep your body in a long line from head to back heel as you move. Complete the repetitions on one leg; then switch legs.

Protocol

Sets: 3-4
Reps: 6-8 each side
Rest: 60 sec

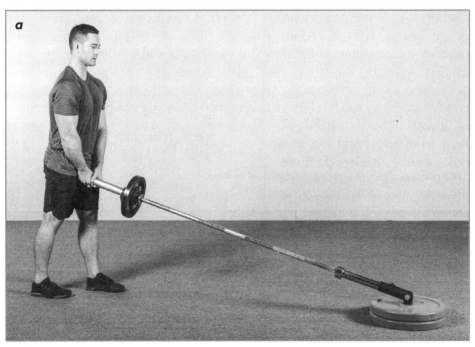

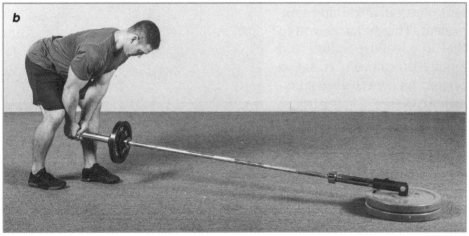

Clearly, the Romanian deadlift is a staple exercise in any great program, and as we begin to increase the difficulty of hip-dominant exercises, the Romanian deadlift will be instrumental in allowing us to increase loading capacity. We also have the ability to include accommodating resistance (AR), which not only provides novelty but can further develop hip hinge mechanics. With any great exercise, there is always the question of how to create variation and consistently allow positive adaptations to occur, but it's also important to consider making improvements in motor patterns, increases in strength gains, and improvements in body composition. An easy tactic is adding relatively inexpensive resistance bands that forcefully pull you forward and add a reactive neuromuscular training component. This requires you to dial in a solid position and engage the anterior core and posterior chain to even greater potential.

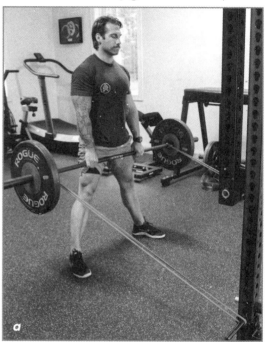

Instructions

- Attach two resistance bands to a fixed object such as a squat rack and then place the other side of the bands around a barbell.
- Stand with your feet wider than hip-width apart, toes slightly pointed out in a sumo stance.
- Hold the barbell in both hands using a clean grip (double overhand, palms facing you) at mid thigh.

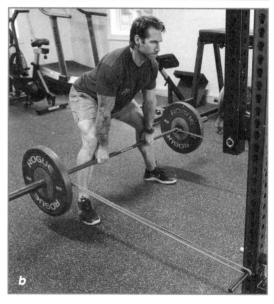

- Step back roughly 8 to 10 inches (20 to 25 cm) until there is full tension on the bands (there should be tension through the entire movement) (see figure *a*).
- Hinge at the hips to lower the barbell toward the floor (see figure *b*). Your hips lead the movement, not your knees. The knees stay unlocked but static.
- Arch your lower back and tuck your chin.
- Engage your abdominals and lats, and resist the band pulling you forward.
- Once you feel a stretch in your hamstrings, reverse the movement to return to the start position. As you reverse position, your lumbar curve should remain intact. (The lower back should have an arch through both the lowering and raising phases of this movement.)

Protocol

Sets: 4-5

Reps: 8-10

Rest: 90 sec to 2 min

Variations

Sumo Stance Romanian Deadlift With Reverse Bands

To perform the sumo stance Romanian deadlift with reverse bands, follow the same mechanics as previously described but two resistance bands will be affixed to the top of your squat rack and then around the collars of your barbell, which will provide an unloading effect on the

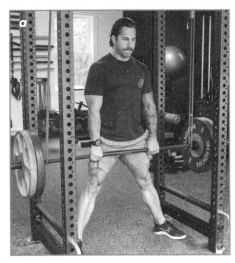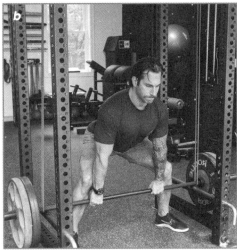

barbell. This variation has the benefit of using AR in reverse—bands applied to the top of your rack, taking load off of the barbell at the start position. The advantage here is to unload the top position to a degree that allows you to start the Romanian deadlift with great movement mechanics (see figure *a*). As you lower and the bands are stretched, the load increases (see figure *b*). This allows for greater levels of trainability with heavier loads without compromising technique. In most cases, reverse bands are a great tool to improve technique.

Protocol
Sets: 4

Reps: 8-10

Rest: 90 sec

Conventional Stance Romanian Deadlift With Bands Pulling Forward

To perform the conventional stance Romanian deadlift with bands pulling forward, follow the same mechanics as previously described, but stand with your feet hip-width apart and toes pointed forward (see figures *a* and *b*).

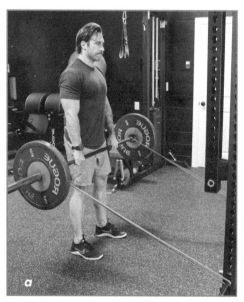
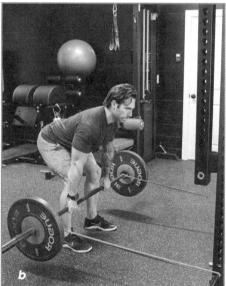

Protocol
Sets: 4

Reps: 8-10

Rest: 90 sec

The Russian kettlebell swing is another exercise to train the hip hinge pattern, but it does so in a dynamic and explosive fashion, making it more difficult than the previous exercises. (The Romanian deadlift pattern is a prerequisite.) Russian kettlebell swings allow you to forcefully train hip extension and athletic ability, and their explosive strength component makes them a great tool to prime the sympathetic nervous system prior to training. (They induce a fight-or-flight response that allows you to be fully prepared for your upcoming training session.)

This exercise can have a wide variety of applications in program design; it can be used optimally for both strength and conditioning, but its application doesn't end there. Russian kettlebell swings can be used as a warm-up tool, as a strength development tool (heavy loads, 8- to 10-rep range), as a strength endurance tool (moderate loads, 12- to 15-rep range), and as a conditioning tool outside of a traditional strength-based session (lighter loads, 15+-rep range).

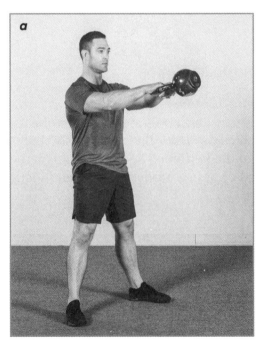
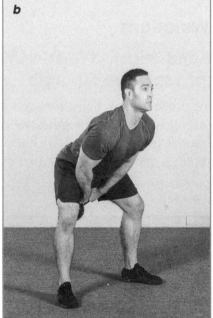

Instructions

- Stand with your feet hip-width apart, abdominals engaged and chin tucked.
- Hold a kettlebell by the handle with both hands, arms straight, to let the kettlebell hang in between your legs.

- Hinge with the hips, bend the knees slightly, and forcefully drive the hips forward to swing the kettlebell until it's at about mid abdomen level in front of you (see figure *a*). Keep the arms straight.
- Your hips lead the movement, not your knees. Your knees stay unlocked but static.
- Squeeze your glutes at the top of the swing.
- As the kettlebell starts to swing back down between the legs, hinge at the hips and slightly bend your knees (see figure *b*).
- Immediately begin the next swing, moving continuously as the kettlebell swings.

Protocol

Sets: 3-4

Reps: 12-15

Rest: 60 sec

Variations

Band-Resisted Russian Kettlebell Swing for Explosive Strength

To perform the band-resisted Russian kettlebell swing for explosive strength, follow the same mechanics as described previously, but a band is looped around the handle of the kettlebell and you stand on the band to secure it (see figures *a* and *b*). Use a moderate load and focus

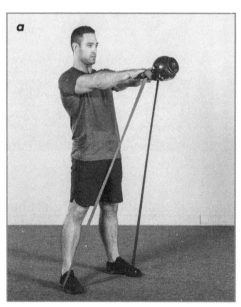
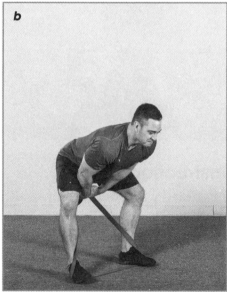

on being explosive with all repetitions—in this context we'll use small, explosive bouts of work with short rest intervals. Affixing a resistance band to the kettlebell and standing on it as the anchor point provides an overspeed eccentric (accentuated lowering phase) and increases the number of activated motor units.

Protocol

Sets: 6
Reps: 3
Rest: 45 sec

Russian Kettlebell Swing for Strength and Hypertrophy Work

To perform the Russian kettlebell swing for strength and hypertrophy work, follow the same mechanics as described previously, but the amount of load will change to roughly 50 percent of your bodyweight. For hypertrophy, use a heavier load, something that will challenge you to perform sets of 10 to 15 reps.

Protocol

Sets: 4
Reps: 10-15
Rest: 90 sec

Russian Kettlebell Swing as a Finisher

To perform the Russian kettlebell swing as a finisher, follow the same mechanics as described previously, using close to or the same load you used for hypertrophy work. The goal here is to perform 100 reps in as few sets as possible.

Protocol

Sets: N/A
Reps: 100 in as few sets as possible
Rest: As little as possible

GLUTE-HAM RAISE

The glute-ham raise is the Cadillac of hamstring exercises, isolating the hamstrings to high degree. With the exercise's level of effectiveness comes a high level of strength requisite—you'll need to be quite strong already to perform this exercise. Glute-ham raises are comparable to Nordic hamstring curls, which isolate the hamstrings through ROM, forcing you to recruit the hamstrings and calves to a high degree on each repetition.

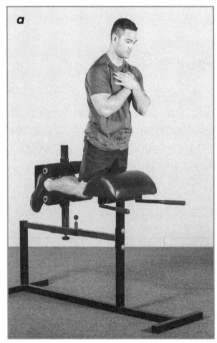
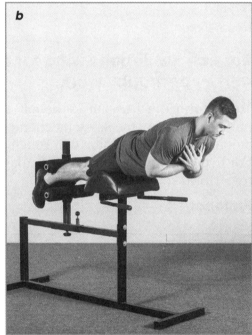

Instructions

- Adjust the glute-ham raise machine so that the bottoms of your thighs are at the bottom of the pad.
- Start with your torso upright and arms crossed over your chest (see figure *a*).
- Lower yourself with control by extending from the knees until your upper body is parallel to the floor (see figure *b*). Keep the lower back rigid.
- Initiate the upward movement to return to the start position by pressing your toes hard against the back plate.

Protocol
Sets: 3-4
Reps: 6-8
Rest: 90 sec

Variations

Hand-Assisted Glute-Ham Raise

The hand-assisted glute-ham raise uses the same set-up, but now you'll position a box in front of the machine that you'll place your hands on and push off from in completing the concentric phase of this movement (see figures *a* and *b*).

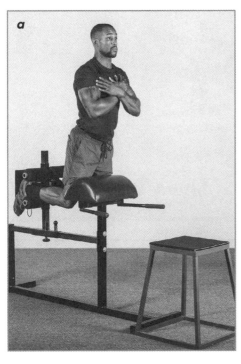
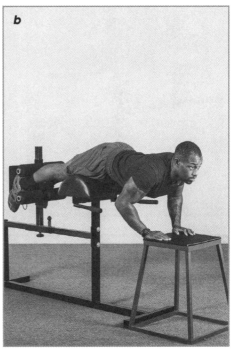

Protocol
Sets: 4
Reps: 4-6
Rest: 90 sec

Band-Assisted Glute-Ham Raise

The band-assisted glute-ham raise uses the same set-up, but now you'll use a band to attach to the back plate of the machine to provide additional assistance for both lowering and raising (see figures *a* and *b*).

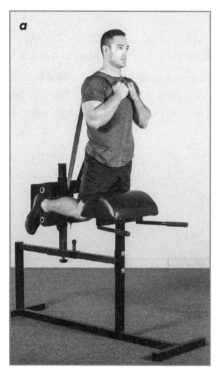
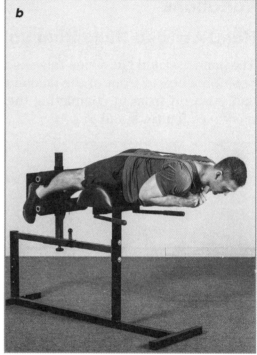

Protocol
Sets: 4
Reps: 5-7
Rest: 90 sec

Loaded Glute-Ham Raise

The loaded glute-ham raise uses the same set-up, but now you'll add load in the form of a weighted vest or medicine ball held anteriorly (see figures *a* and *b*).

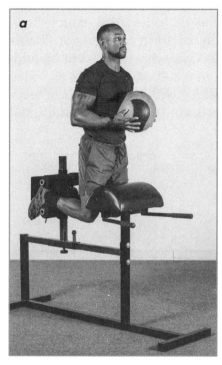
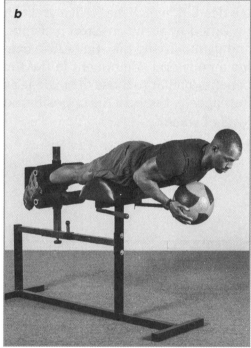

Protocol
Sets: 4
Reps: 6-8
Rest: 90 sec

The trap bar deadlift is an excellent hip hinge exercise because using the trap bar rather than a straight bar brings the load closer to your center of mass, thus creating a completely different gravity line and bar path. This makes the trap bar more user-friendly for those with lower back issues. I've found that far more individuals experience success with the trap bar, improving strength and longevity versus the straight bar deadlift, which makes it a great choice. Of course, this exercise can be varied by using assisted resistance in the form of bands or chains and by modifying the stance. We can also vary this movement by adding a unilateral component in the form of a split stance; this provides benefits similar to those of single-leg training with higher levels of loading capacity because the opposite (nonworking) leg adds an additional level of stability.

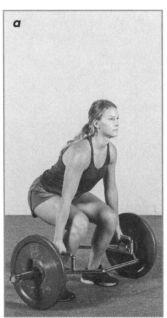 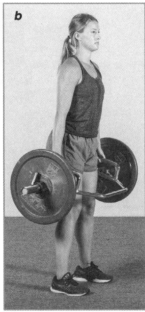 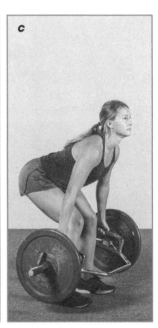

Instructions

- Stand inside the trap bar with your feet hip-width apart. Bend your knees to lower your hips, and grasp the trap bar with each hand (see figure *a*).
- Lift your chest, engage your abdominals, and lift the bar off the ground by extending your knees until you are standing upright (see figure *b*).
- Hinge at your hips, slightly bend your knees, and arch your back as you lower the bar toward the floor (see figure *c*).

- Your hips lead the movement, not your knees. Your knees stay unlocked but static.
- Lower to the floor until both plates are touching the ground—this is 1 rep.
- Each repetition starts on the ground.

Protocol
Sets: 5
Reps: Build to a heavy 5 or 5RM
Rest: 2-3 min

Variations

Trap Bar Romanian Deadlift

The trap bar Romanian deadlift is an excellent hip hinge exercise variation to execute the often-forgotten hip hinge pattern. The trap bar deadlift pulls the load from the floor, while this movement starts in the top position and the repetition starts with the eccentric (lowering phase) (see figures *a* and *b*). While this variation does not carry the same loading capacity as its trap bar deadlift counterpart, it is an excellent variation to reinforce hip hinging mechanics and train the hamstrings group to a high degree.

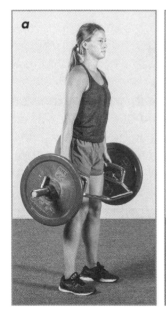
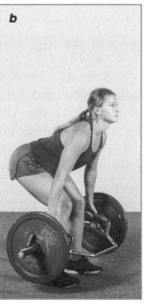

Protocol
Sets: 4
Reps: 8-10
Rest: 90 sec to 2 min

Split Stance Trap Bar Romanian Deadlift

The split stance trap bar Romanian deadlift is performed with the same set-up and execution as the trap bar RDL, except that one leg is staggered 3 to 4 inches (8 to 10 cm) behind the other (see figures *a* and *b*).

Protocol
Sets: 4
Reps: 6-8 each side
Rest: 90 sec

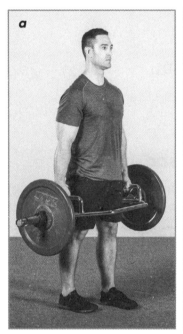
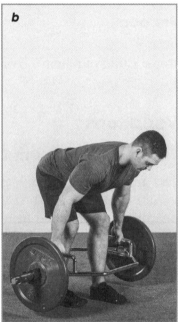

Trap Bar Romanian Deadlift With Band Pulling Forward

The trap bar Romanian deadlift with band pulling forward is executed in the same manner as the trap bar RDL, except that one band is affixed to a squat rack or a heavy fixed object in front of you (see figures *a* and *b*). The band pulling forward will force you to engage your anterior core and lats to a great degree and provide a new challenge to a foundational movement pattern.

Protocol
Sets: 4
Reps: 8-10
Rest: 90 sec

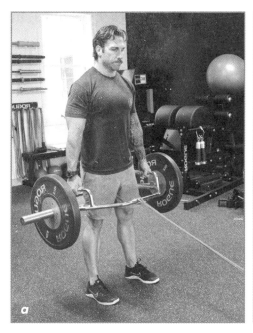
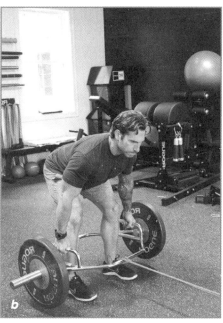

Trap Bar Deadlift Clusters

To perform trap bar deadlift clusters, perform the prescribed number of repetitions and rest between each cluster set. For example, for a cluster set of 3.2.1 (15 seconds), perform 3 trap bar deadlifts and after your third rep, lower the weight and rest 15 seconds before performing your next set of 2. Perform 2 repetitions and then rest again for 15 seconds. Finally, perform your final repetition and then rest for 3 minutes.

Protocol
Sets: 3
Reps: 3.2.1 (15 sec) @ 80%-85% of 1RM
Rest: 3 min

SUMO STANCE RACK DEADLIFT

At the top of the skill pyramid we find sumo stance rack deadlifts. In this exercise, we're elevating the sumo stance deadlift off the floor by using a rack or simply elevating the plates on mats. Decreasing the ROM of the sumo stance deadlift encourages spinal neutrality and optimizes loading capacity. Key here is that a neutral spine is maintained. The rack makes this exercise easier to customize to the individual based on anthropometrics, training history, and training age. While many will be able to achieve potential loads that exceed their current one-repetition maximum with decreased ROM, the objective here is to maintain optimal positioning, *not* just loading capacity. It's important to note that the sumo stance rack deadlift can be used both in a heavy maximal setting with the maximal effort (ME) or submaximal effort method as a main lift (first lift in your session) and in a speed-based dynamic effort (DE) session; these protocols are listed here. The former (ME and submaximal effort) is geared at

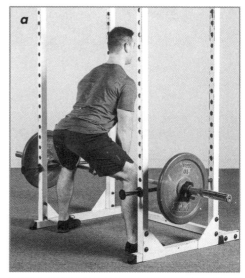

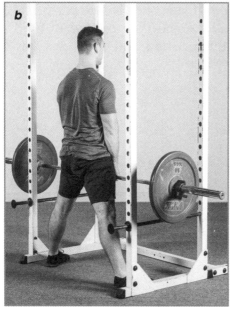

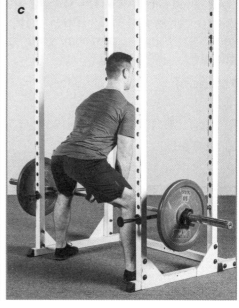

maximal strength development by working the force portion of the force-velocity curve, while the latter (DE) improves rate of force development by working the velocity portion of the force-velocity curve.

Instructions

- Set the barbell in the rack so that it's at mid shin height.
- Stand with your feet wider than hip-width apart and toes pointed slightly out. Hinge at the hips and bend your knees slightly to reach down for the bar (see figure *a*).
- Grasp the barbell in both hands using a clean grip (double overhand, palms facing you) or a mixed grip (one overhand, one underhand).
- Arch your lower back, tuck your chin, and engage your abdominals and lats.
- Pull the bar up as you extend your knees and shift your hips forward to stand up (see figure *b*). Squeeze your glutes at the top.
- Hinge at the hips to lower the weight until you feel a stretch in your hamstrings (see figure *c*). Your hips lead the movement, not your knees. Your knees stay unlocked but static.

Protocol

Sets: 8
Reps: Build to a 1RM
Rest: 3 min

Variations

Sumo Stance Deadlift Against a Band

The sumo stance deadlift against a band is executed in the same manner as the sumo stance rack deadlift, except that the barbell is not in a rack and a band is positioned over the bar to utilize AR. Set up in your stance with the band draped over the bar, and stand on the band with both feet (see figures *a* and *b*).

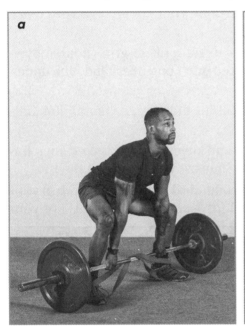
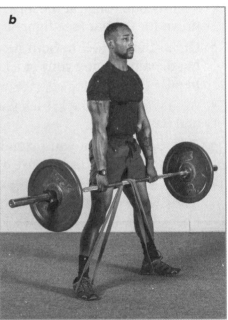

Protocol

Sets: 6
Reps: 3RM
Rest: 3 min

Sumo Stance Deadlift Against a Band for Dynamic Effort

The sumo stance deadlift against a band for dynamic effort is executed in the same manner as the sumo stance rack deadlift, except that the barbell is not in a rack and a band is positioned over the bar to utilize AR. Set up in your stance with the band draped over the bar, and stand on the band with both feet. (You are the anchor point.) Use light loads and perform repetitions with focus on being explosive and aggressive with each repetition while still using correct positioning.

Protocol
Sets: 6
Reps: 2 @ 50% of 1RM + band tension
Rest: 60 sec

In short, hip-dominant exercises are arguably the most important aspect of the majority of training plans we write, and the logic is simple. It's worth saying again that the large majority of the population is plagued with lower back pain, some if not most of which can be attributed to lack of strength in supporting musculature such as the hamstrings and glutes. This musculature does not take a back seat to any other muscle groups and is a mainstay in any great training plan.

Chapter 7

Isolation Exercises

Anyone training for aesthetics is likely familiar with a long list of isolation exercises, but over the last decade isolation exercises have become less popular in favor of larger foundational patterns like squats and hinge variations. Performing foundational patterns is arguably the more important aspect of a great program. At the same time, I'd challenge you to consider that you're only as strong as your weakest link, and using isolation exercises to strategically improve deficits will not only improve foundational patterns but also prevent injury and add lean mass to lagging muscle groups. While you can simply continue to safely add volume to multijoint movements forever, there comes a point of diminishing returns. Isolation exercises offer a bridge between multijoint and single-joint exercises where you can increase strength without necessarily increasing the risk of mechanical breakdown.

Before we look at the exercises, here are a few things to consider regarding exercise selection and volume prescription for optimal isolation exercise programming for the lower body.

EXERCISE SELECTION

Every exercise in your program should have a clear and concise *why* behind its selection, and in the case of isolation exercises, you should have two goals. The first is to identify the specific purpose of the exercise, and the second is to determine how that exercise assists you in terms of development. For example, let's assume an aspiring CrossFit athlete continuously misses hip extension in their Olympic lifts. Their coach has determined that lack of strength in the gluteus maximus may be the culprit, as they also tend to present sticking points above parallel in the squat and lockout and in the deadlift. Upon further investigation, the athlete tells the coach they cannot "feel" their glutes in glute bridge exercises because their hamstrings tend to predominate in the movement. To remedy this, the coach includes more isolation exercises for the glutes that work the glutes through all functions, including hip extension (bodyweight bridges and thrusts), abduction (hinged-back banded abduction), and external rotation (band-resisted glute bridge). Within eight weeks, the athlete presents better hip extension in their Olympic lifts.

Simple tactics like this have been used for decades, and in fact, some of the strongest athletes in the world are masters of understanding where they are weakest and artists when it comes to inventing new ways to minimize these limitations. Isolation exercises are an integral part of this quest to minimize your limitations, and thus no program is complete without them.

VOLUME PRESCRIPTION

Isolation exercises work for smaller muscle groups, and since the range of motion (ROM) is smaller and the demand on the musculature system is generally lower (think how bilateral movement presents higher demands on larger muscle groups than unilateral movement), you can safely perform high-volume sets with less chance of creating compensation patterns. For example, if someone trying to develop the lockout of their bench press selected a close-grip bench press as an assistance exercise followed by a triceps pushdown, the latter exercise is far less demanding, making it more realistic to perform in high-volume work sets. For areas of the body like the hamstrings or glute complex, opt for higher rep ranges. Additionally, considering the breakdown of muscle fiber types of each muscle group can provide further guidance as to what rep ranges will be more suitable. For example, the glute complex responds quite well to higher rep schemes such as 15+ because it is made up of slower-twitch type I muscle fiber, whereas the hamstrings respond very well to lower-rep schemes due to their high concentration of fast-twitch muscle fiber. Because isolation exercises are better able to isolate a lagging muscle group, prescribing high doses of volume is not only safe but quite effective. Above all else, the volume, exercise selection, and frequency within a program should align with your limitations, goals, and needs.

We know that many people exhibit weaknesses in their glutes, hamstrings, and general posterior musculature. Our daily postures are certainly not helping these limitations and only exacerbate these weaknesses. The good news is that we can target these weaker muscle groups with simple exercises geared at isolating the musculature of the lower body.

Band Training

We've spent the majority of this book discussing optimal means of training for the lower body via the barbell, dumbbells, and tools like accommodating resistance (AR). Performing high-volume resistance band work has many advantages. For instance, this work directly aids in strengthening connective tissue, which will help prevent potential soft-tissue injuries. Another benefit is greater storage of kinetic energy via the series elastic component (SEC), which includes muscular components, although tendons constitute the majority of it. When stretched during eccentric ROM, the SEC acts as a spring, which correlates to higher reversible strength (ability to go from eccentric to concentric contractions), thus improving the explosive strength capability of an athlete (Potach and Chu 2016). Included in our list of isolation exercises are many that include the use of bands, so it makes sense to explain why bands are beneficial based on the physiology behind their inclusion in this book. Here are some of the benefits of bands:

- Bands can be used for high amounts of work with little risk of injury or delayed onset muscle soreness (DOMS), which is a bonus if you're trying to perform more work and not take away from your main training sessions.
- For those with lower training ages, movements using bands will help give you the experience to improve your mind-muscle connection, making it easy for you to feel the correct musculature working.
- Bands improve tendon elasticity and increase stored kinetic energy in tendons because they facilitate high-volume, rapid repetitions.
- Bands create hypertrophic adaptations and the ability of the muscles to generate more force, thereby increasing your overall strength.
- Bands are highly effective when used in your warm-up sequence to prepare you for an upcoming training session. Variations have a multitude of uses and are not just for "finishers."
- Bands are incredibly easy to teach and perform, making them a great option for your clients if you're a trainer.

(continued)

Band Training *(continued)*

It is also important to understand the differences between bands and cables and the purpose of each. Both band work and cable work are an integral part of any program; they are similar but serve different purposes, as follows:

- Bands are a form of AR (tension increases through ROM), whereas cables provide constant tension through ROM.
- Bands work better for high-volume sets (25 to 50 reps, for example), whereas cables work best in a hypertrophy setting (12 to 30 reps, for example).

While bands are simply another training tool, they can be a game changer for those who are not currently using them. You'll see more than a few exercises in this chapter that include the use of bands.

LATERAL SLED DRAG

The unilateral nature of the sled and its ability to train the lower body without high amounts of tissue breakdown make the sled a great fit for isolating specific patterns and muscles (in this case the adductors and the gluteus medius). Moreover, training in the frontal plane is often neglected, which presents an area of opportunity to create more balance in your programming. We often talk about training in the sagittal plane (think squats and deadlifts), but the frontal plane is an area of low-hanging fruit for many, and a great place to start is with this simple lateral sled drag.

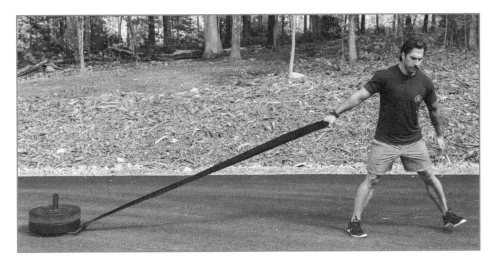

Instructions
- Stand in front of the sled and grab its straps in your right hand.
- Turn so that your right side faces the sled and assume an athletic stance with your feet hip-width apart and a slight bend in the knees.
- Hold straps at hip level.
- Pull the sled forward by performing a side-step action, stepping to the left about 10 to 12 inches (25 to 30 cm) with the left foot, and then following with the right foot to come back into a hip-width stance (see figure).
- Continue until you've covered the distance; then switch sides so that your left side faces the sled and you lead with the right foot.

Protocol
Sets: 6
Reps: 30 yd (27 m) each side
Rest: 60-90 sec

Variation

Lateral Sled Drag Carioca

To perform a lateral sled drag carioca, follow the same mechanics as described previously, but your legs will cross over each other on each step (see figure): step to the side with the left foot, and then bring the right foot in front of the left foot and place it on the ground to the outside of the left foot. Continue until you've covered the distance; then switch sides so that your left side faces the sled and you lead with the right foot.

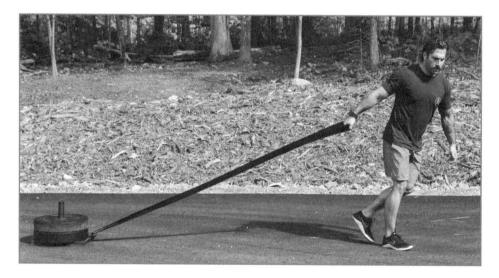

Protocol

Sets: 6
Reps: 30 yd (27 m) each side
Rest: 60-90 sec

SINGLE-LEG DUMBBELL CALF RAISE

The single-leg calf raise is a great exercise to train the calf through a full ROM, through both plantar flexion and dorsiflexion. Here, we use a dumbbell for resistance as a simple way to isolate the calf muscles, in particular the gastrocnemius, which has a high concentration of fast-twitch muscle fiber. The calves respond well to high-volume training and slow and controlled repetitions because they already sustain high amounts of volume daily as you move around. In order to provide a noteworthy stimulus to the calves to promote growth, you need to consider using high-volume techniques over time (after you have become accustomed to regular calf training) and high frequency (the number of sessions that include direct calf work on a weekly basis). It's important to note that calf growth is highly genetic in terms of size. I've seen many individuals struggle to add size to their calves despite using the best training practices on a weekly basis, so it's important to set realistic goals when training this area.

Instructions

- Stand with the feet hip-width apart. Grasp a dumbbell in the hand on the side of the working leg. If you choose, you may stand on a platform or box to add 1 to 2 inches (2.5 to 5 cm) of elevation for extra ROM.
- Shift your weight slightly to the working leg (see figure *a*).
- Fully extend the foot of the working leg, lifting the heel off the floor, and pause, balancing on the ball of your foot for 1 count (see figure *b*).
- Lower under control, pausing for 1 count at the bottom.
- Complete the repetitions on one leg; then move the dumbbell to the other hand and perform on the other leg.

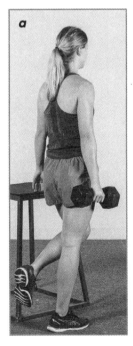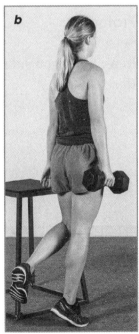

Protocol
Sets: 3-4
Reps: 8-10 each side
Rest: 60 sec

Variation

1-1/4 Single-Leg Dumbbell Calf Raise

The benefit of the 1-1/4 single-leg dumbbell calf raise is that it adds time under tension to the calf raise, which is particularly advantageous for those with stubborn calf muscles in regard to growth. Much like other 1-1/4 variations in this book, you'll perform the movement with an extra quarter rep at the top of the movement. Perform a full single-leg calf raise and once you are at the top of the movement (end ROM), go back down only a quarter of the way and then back up to the end ROM (see figures *a-d*). This constitutes 1 rep.

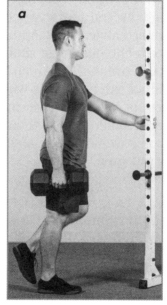
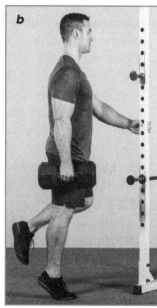
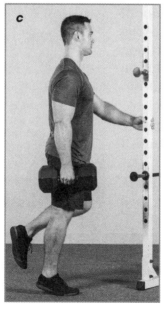
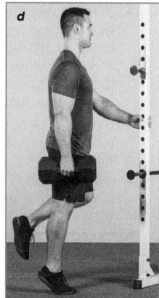

Protocol

Sets: 3-4
Reps: 8-10 each side
Rest: 60 sec

PLATE-LOADED CALF RAISE

The plate-loaded calf raise is a great exercise to train the calves bilaterally for higher-repetition sets. Using a dip belt is an excellent way to train strength endurance qualities of the calf muscles with more emphasis on the soleus, which presents more slow-twitch muscle fiber. Sets of 15+ reps are in line for this exercise, with repetitions being more rapid compared to those of its slower and more controlled counterpart, the single-leg dumbbell calf raise.

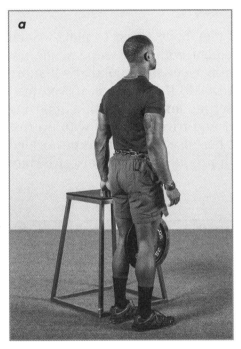
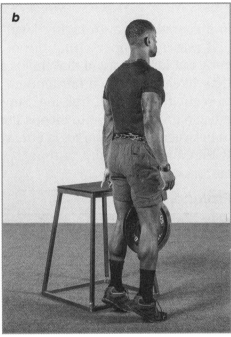

Instructions

- Place the dip belt around your waist and adjust the length of the chain as needed. Attach a weight plate to the belt so that it hangs in a comfortable position for you—likely somewhere between the knees and the groin. Use a weight that allows you to perform at least 15 repetitions without stopping.
- Stand with your feet hip-width or slightly wider apart, and place a hand on a fixed object for support (see figure *a*).
- Lift both heels off the floor as you perform repetitions explosively and fully extend your legs, flexing the calves at the top of each repetition (see figure *b*).
- You will go up to the balls of the feet on each rep and down to the heels when you lower.

Protocol
Sets: 3-4
Reps: 12-15
Rest: 60 sec

Variation

Plate-Loaded Calf Raise Supersets

You can add an even higher level of metabolic stress to plate-loaded calf raises by supersetting the movement with jump rope single unders, but keep in mind that this is an advanced protocol that will more than likely result in a fair amount of DOMS if you're not accustomed to regular direct calf training. Supersetting involves training opposing muscle groups, e.g., the biceps group and triceps group, with no rest in between. This superset is effective because its volume is performed within a short amount of time, which produces high levels of lactate and muscle acidity.

Protocol
Sets: 3-4
Reps: 12-15
Rest: 60 sec

The barbell tibia raise + calf raise is a bilateral exercise that includes a tibia raise (toe raise) before the calf raise. The advantage of adding the tibia raise is added stress to the tibialis anterior, which when developed can make the calves appear larger. When considering how to increase loading capacity for the calves, barbell variations usually come to mind. While the exercises earlier in this chapter have their place in any great training program, adding loading capacity in the form of dumbbells or a loaded dip belt has its limitations. Using a barbell increases the loading capability, adding another dimension to your training. If you've never performed a traditional barbell calf raise before, I'd recommend starting with that variation and advancing to the tibia raise + calf raise variation when you're ready.

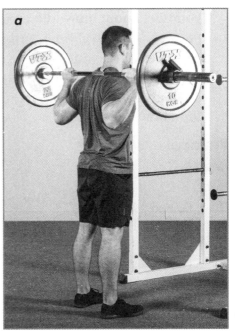

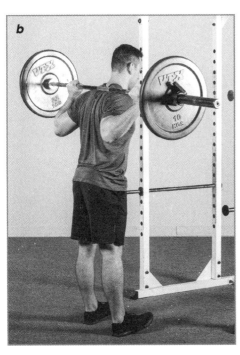

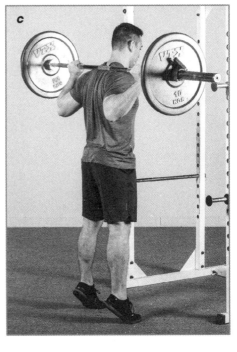

Instructions

- Set your barbell up in a squat rack.
- Position the barbell on your back over the mid traps and place your feet about hip-width apart (see figure *a*).
- Perform a tibia raise by lifting your toes off the floor and placing your weight on your heels (see figure *b*).
- Return your toes to the floor and lift your heels to place your weight on your toes (see figure *c*). Fully extend and flex the calves at the top of the movement.

Protocol

Sets: 4

Reps: 8-10

Rest: 60 sec

Variation

Barbell Calf Raise

The barbell calf raise is a bilateral exercise performed with the barbell placed on your upper traps (the same position you'd hold the barbell in if you were performing a back squat) and with feet shoulder-width apart, then completing a bilateral calf raise. Much like other variations listed, this variation is performed with a slow and controlled concentric and eccentric phase to bypass the stretch-shortening cycle that the calves are accustomed to utilizing (see figures *a* and *b*).

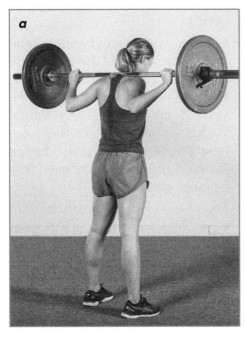 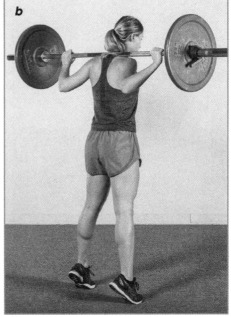

Protocol

Sets: 4
Reps: 8-10
Rest: 60 sec

The seated single-leg banded hamstring curl effectively isolates the hamstrings as well as improves the strength and abilities of tendons, making it a great exercise to include in your program. Clearly, the hamstrings are a muscle group that requires a fair amount of attention for weekend warriors and athletes alike, and using bands is an incredible way to target these fast-twitch-dominant muscles. The banded hamstring curl can be performed both unilaterally and bilaterally; the following instructions work one leg at a time.

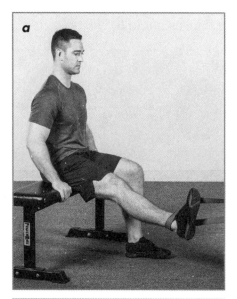

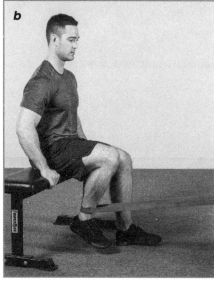

Instructions

- Sit on a standard 16-inch (40 cm) bench.
- Loop a resistance band behind your leg just above the ankle, and attach the ends of the band to a fixed object in front of you. When you extend your leg, there should be light resistance on the band (see figure *a*); move the bench forward or back if you need less or more resistance.
- From the seated position with your leg extended, flex your knee and pull your foot toward you so that the foot goes under the bench (see figure *b*). There should be tension throughout your full ROM.
- Quickly return the leg to the extended position to complete 1 rep.
- Complete the reps on one leg; then switch legs.

Protocol

Sets: 5
Reps: 25 each side
Rest: As needed

Variations

Seated Banded Hamstring Curl for Activation

To perform the seated banded hamstring curl for activation, follow the same mechanics as described previously, but the amount of resistance will change. In this case, use a light band—something you could easily perform sets of 8 to 10 slow and controlled reps with.

Protocol

Sets: 3
Reps: 8-10 each side
Rest: 60 sec

Seated Banded Hamstring Curl as a Finisher

To perform the seated banded hamstring curl as a finisher, follow the same mechanics as described previously, but the amount of resistance will change. In this case, use the same band as for activation (light band) but with higher volume and higher frequency of repetitions.

Protocol

Sets: 3
Reps: 50 each side
Rest: 60 sec

The bilateral version of the seated banded hamstring curl comes with the same benefits as its single-leg counterpart, but performing the exercise with both legs increases the band thickness required to provide the tension for this variation to be effective (usually a band that is double the thickness of its single-leg counterpart).

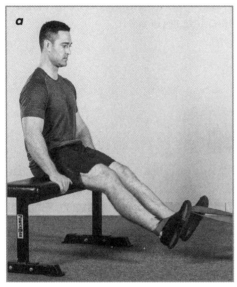
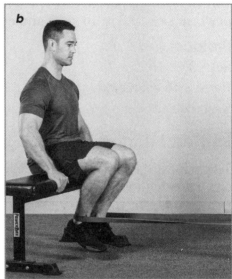

Instructions

- Sit on a standard 16-inch (40 cm) bench.
- Loop a resistance band behind both of your legs just above the ankles, and attach the ends of the band to a fixed object in front of you. When you extend your legs, there should be light resistance on the band (see figure *a*); move the bench forward or back if you need less or more resistance.
- From the seated position with both legs extended, flex your knees and pull your feet toward you so that the feet go under the bench (see figure *b*). There should be tension throughout your full ROM.
- Quickly return the legs to the extended position to complete 1 rep.

Protocol

Sets: 4
Reps: 20-30
Rest: 60 sec

Variations

Seated Double-Leg Banded Hamstring Curl for Activation

To perform the seated double-leg banded hamstring curl for activation, follow the same mechanics as described previously. Since this movement is performed bilaterally, you'll likely be able to handle using a heavy-resistance band, but perform the exercise now with more of a slow and controlled tempo.

Protocol

Sets: 3
Reps: 8-10
Rest: 60 sec

Seated Double-Leg Banded Hamstring Curl as a High-Volume Finisher

This variation's major difference now lies in the execution. Using the same band thickness as for the seated double-leg banded hamstring curl, repetitions will be performed with a higher cycle rate as the goal is to create more metabolic stress whereas for activation the intent was to simply prepare for the upcoming training where massive amounts of volume are not necessary.

Protocol

Sets: 4
Reps: 25
Rest: 60 sec

BAND-RESISTED GLUTE BRIDGE

The band-resisted glute bridge is another exercise that uses AR for added difficulty and activation of key muscles—in this case, the glute complex. Like the banded hamstrings curls, this exercise can be used both in a warm-up sequence and as a finishing isolation exercise. It also helps to increase mind-muscle connection, which is particularly advantageous if you have trouble feeling your glutes work. As band tension increases at end of ROM, it allows you to forcefully contract the glutes so that you can feel them work. (It's common for people to report not feeling their glutes working with nonbanded bridge variations—there are a number of reasons for this that are unique to individuals.)

Instructions

- Start in a supine position with your knees bent, a band secured under both heels, and the loop of the band placed over the bottom of your thighs (see figure *a*). Keep your heels on the ground so the band doesn't lose tension. The foot placement can be customized based on your anthropometrics. For example, if you feel this exercise only in your hamstrings rather than in your glutes, try moving your feet closer to your glutes.

- Push down into your heels and lift your hips off the floor, creating a fulcrum at the upper back. Fully extend your hips and pause to squeeze the glutes at the top of the movement (see figure *b*).

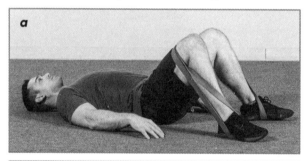

- Reverse the movement to lower your hips to the floor.

Protocol
Sets: 3
Reps: 8-10
Rest: 60 sec

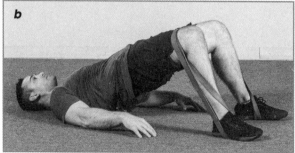

Variations

Band-Resisted Glute Bridge for Activation

To perform the band-resisted glute bridge for activation, follow the same mechanics as described previously, but add a 2-second isometric hold at the top of each rep to ensure full contraction of the glute complex.

Protocol

Sets: 3

Reps: 5, with 2 sec holds at top

Rest: 60 sec

Band-Resisted Glute Bridge as a Finisher

To perform the band-resisted glute bridge as a finisher, follow the same mechanics as described previously, but perform all repetitions in more of a constant cadence with no pauses at the bottom or the top.

Protocol

Sets: 4

Reps: 12-15

Rest: 60 sec

The lying hamstring leg curl requires a lying leg curl machine, which is a great piece of equipment. This is an excellent variation to isolate the hamstrings, similar to the glute-ham raise introduced in chapter 6 but more user-friendly in that you can adjust the resistance based on your ability. Moreover, this exercise works well using heavier loads because the hamstrings are composed of predominantly fast-twitch muscle fiber. Many people make the mistake of programming higher-rep schemes, but taking the opposite approach will elicit better results. This exercise can be performed both bilaterally and unilaterally.

Instructions

- Lie face down (prone) on the lying leg curl machine and place the backs of your ankles under the padded bar (see figure *a*).

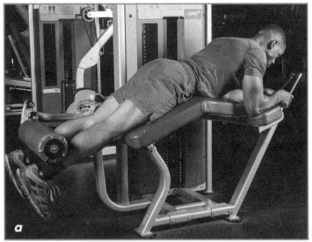

- Hold the handles to anchor your body.
- Initiate the movement by flexing at the knees, using your hamstrings to bring your feet toward your body (see figure *b*).
- Point your toes to the floor at the top and then return to the start position by extending your knees.

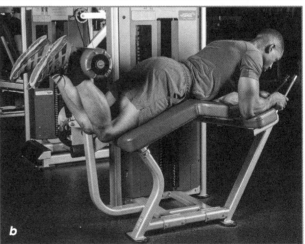

Protocol
Sets: 4
Reps: 8-10
Rest: 90 sec

Variation

Single-Leg Lying Hamstring Leg Curl

To perform the single-leg lying hamstring leg curl, follow the same mechanics as described previously, but place just one leg under the padded bar.

Protocol

Sets: 4
Reps: 6-8 each side
Rest: 60 sec

The seated calf raise is a great exercise and a common piece of equipment for any commercial gym. Your calf muscles consist primarily of two components: the gastrocnemius and the soleus. The seated calf raise allows for high levels of metabolic stress on the soleus, which is composed of more slow-twitch muscle fiber than the gastrocnemius. This means you can perform a high volume of reps per set. To elicit even higher levels of metabolic stress and not use the stretch-shortening cycle, add a slight pause between repetitions.

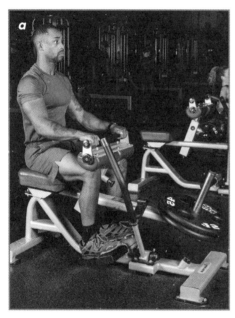 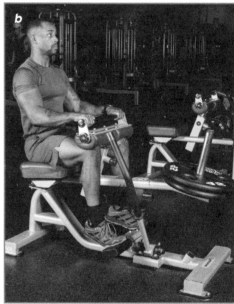

Instructions

- Sit on the pad of the seated calf raise machine, selecting a load that will allow you to perform 12 to 15 repetitions. Place your feet on the foot bar or platform with your knees under the knee pads (see figure *a*).
- Raise your heels as you extend and flex your calves at the top of each rep (see figure *b*).
- Lower your heels and get a full stretch of the calves at the bottom of each rep.

Protocol

Sets: 3
Reps: 12-15
Rest: 60 sec

Variation

Seated Calf Raise 21s

To perform seated calf raise 21s, use the same mechanics as described previously, but in cluster sets of 3 minisets of 7 reps (3 × 7 = 21). The idea is that quick bouts of rest between minisets (in this case 7 reps) will allow you to perform higher amounts of volume per set. In this variation, you'll perform 7 reps, rack the weight and rest 15 seconds, unrack the weight and perform another 7 reps, rerack the weight and rest 15 seconds, and finally perform the final miniset of 7 reps before resting 2 minutes between sets.

Protocol

Sets: 3
Reps: 7.7.7 (15 sec)
Rest: 2 min

SINGLE-LEG HINGED-BACK BANDED ABDUCTION

The single-leg hinged-back banded abduction is an exercise performed in your warm-up sequence to activate the glutes. While we've covered other hip extension exercises for the glute complex, this one places more stress on the gluteus medius, which is responsible for hip abduction—a vital glute function. This exercise includes stability work as well as improving abduction motor patterns, which makes it a good choice for a warm-up.

Instructions

- Stand with the feet about hip-width apart and a light-resistance mini band placed just above your knees.
- Hinge at the hips to push your hips back behind you, with your lower back arched, your chest over your bent knees, and your chin tucked (see figure *a*). This is the start position.
- Using your outer hips (the gluteus medius), open up your legs into abduction while maintaining balance on one leg (see figure *b*). Think of opening up the knees like you do in a fire hydrant drill.
- Return to the start position.
- Complete the reps on one leg; then switch legs.

Protocol
Sets: 3
Reps: 5 each side
Rest: 60 sec

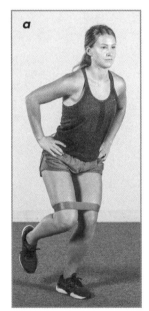
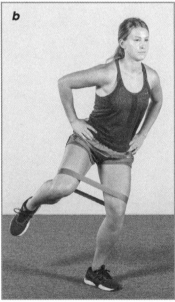

Variation

Single-Leg Hinged-Back Banded Abduction With Support

This variation is a regression of the previous counterpart. Oftentimes individuals have trouble with the balance component, so adding slight support (holding on to a squat rack) will improve balance and allow for more effective abduction movement and thus more recruitment of the gluteus medius. To perform this variation, hold on to a fixed object like a squat rack with the arm of the nonworking side.

Protocol

Sets: 3
Reps: 5 each side
Rest: 60 sec

The seated banded leg extension is an effective tool for training and isolating the quadriceps complex without using an actual leg extension machine. The band does not place the same amount of stress on the patellar tendon, so if you have preexisting knee issues, using a band is likely a better option.

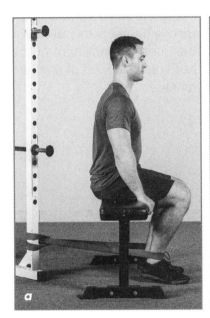 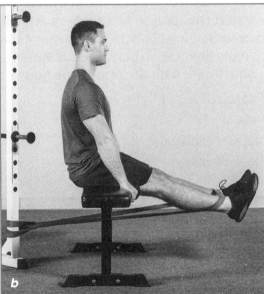

Instructions

- Sit on a bench with a band looped around your ankles and attached to a fix object behind you (see figure *a*).
- Extend your legs and contract your quadriceps at the top of the repetition, when the legs are straight (see figure *b*).
- With control, flex your knees to return to the start position.

Protocol
Sets: 3
Reps: 12-15
Rest: 60 sec

Variation

Seated Banded Single-Leg Extension

To perform the seated banded single-leg extension, use the same mechanics as previously described, but perform with one leg at a time. Performing this exercise unilaterally allows you to train the imbalances in each leg in isolation.

Protocol

Sets: 3
Reps: 8-10 each side
Rest: 60 sec

The barbell glute hip thrust (see chapter 6) is a great exercise to target the glute complex, and its band-resisted counterpart is actually a better fit for some in order to achieve the full benefits of the hip thrust. This is because many people are not used to training the glutes in a hip thrust pattern; also, because so many spend the majority of their lives sitting, they tend to have "glute amnesia" (McGill 2015).

Instructions

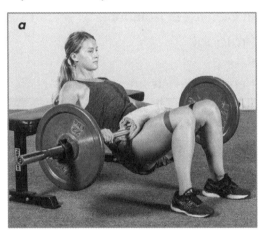

- Sit on the floor in front of the long side of a standard-height weight bench with a light-resistance mini band placed just above your knees.
- Place a standard barbell with a pad or folded towel over your pelvis.
- Raise your body to place your mid back fully on the bench. Place your feet about hip-width apart, and lift your hips until they are close to parallel to the floor.

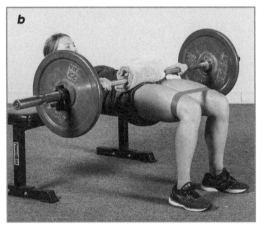

- Start by lowering your hips until your backside is about 1 to 2 inches (2.5 to 5 cm) above the floor. Both legs remain at about 90-degree angles throughout the movement (see figure *a*).
- Push through the heels to initiate upward motion and use the glutes to thrust the hips upward until they are parallel to the floor (see figure *b*). Tuck your chin and squeeze your glutes at the top. That is 1 rep.

Protocol

Sets: 3-4
Reps: 12-15
Rest: 60 sec

Variation

1-1/4 Banded Glute Hip Thrust

The benefits of hip thrusts lie in their ability to effectively train hip extension and in essence all action of the glute complex, but some may need to take a step back because the mind-muscle connection is the linchpin. This variation is beneficial because it uses an additional quarter rep to give a time under tension component. It works best as an assistance exercise on a lower body day, in particular a session that emphasizes the hip hinge pattern. Band resistance allows you to have modified tension, where resistance is highest at end ROM of each rep instead of being constant as with a barbell. For this reason, you may find that you're able to really feel your glutes work each repetition.

For 1-1/4 banded glute hip thrust, use the same mechanics as described previously, but once a full ROM is achieved, perform a quarter rep by going down only a quarter of the way, then going back up to the top of the movement (see figures *a-d*). That is 1 rep.

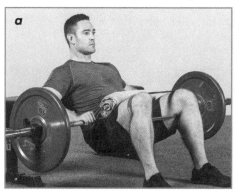
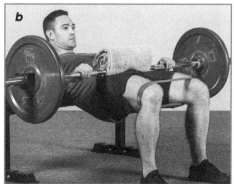
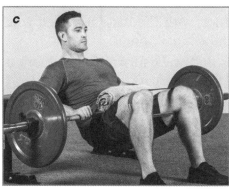
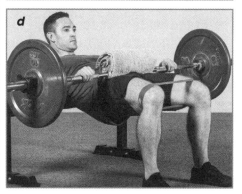

Protocol
Sets: 3
Reps: 12-15 (1 full ROM rep + 1/4 rep at the top of each rep = 1 rep)
Rest: 60 sec

BANDED PULL-THROUGH

The banded pull-through is a great exercise to target the glutes and hamstrings. It can have a multitude of purposes within your programming, such as an activation drill or a high-volume finisher. Although we've talked about the cable pull-through already (see chapter 6), the banded version allows a difference in tension through ROM (i.e., cable tension is constant; band tension is variable). The banded pull-through is for higher training volume with less chance of the onset of local muscle fatigue before each set is complete; in this case, one could go as high as 40 to 50 repetitions per set.

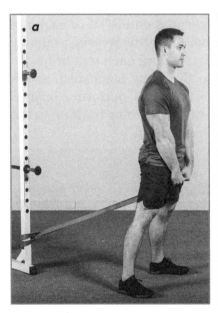
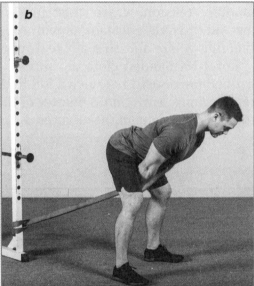

Instructions

- Stand with your feet close together, with the band between your legs, facing away from the band attachment point.
- Grasp the band with both hands and walk forward until there is tension and no slack in the band (see figure *a*).
- Hinge at your hips and bend the knees slightly as you allow your hands to move back behind you (see figure *b*). Think of sitting back, not down. Your hips lead the movement, not your knees; the knees stay unlocked but static.
- Arch your lower back and tuck your chin.
- Once you feel a stretch in your hamstrings to indicate you're at the end of your ROM, reverse the movement by squeezing the glutes to return to standing.

Protocol

Sets: 4
Reps: 25+
Rest: 60 sec

Variation

Banded Pull-Through With Wide Stance

To perform this variation, use the same mechanics as described previously, but assume a wide stance. The wide stance stresses the hips and adductors to a higher degree than the close stance.

Protocol

Sets: 4
Reps: 25+
Rest: 60 sec

The X-band walk + banded good morning is another activation drill for activating the glutes prior to your training session. It can also be used as a high-volume finisher. This exercise trains the glutes via abduction, adduction, and hip extension.

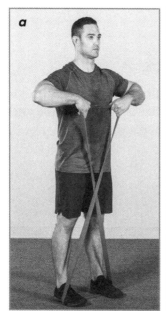
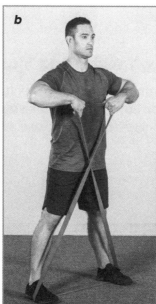
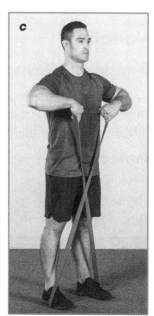
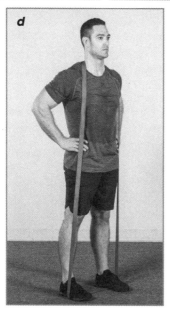
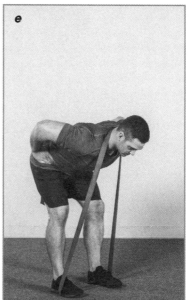

Instructions

- Place a medium-resistance band under both feet, with feet about hip-width apart.

- Twist the band so it forms an X.
- Pull the band upward so there is tension (see figure *a*).
- Step to the left about 8 to 12 inches (20 to 30 cm) with the left foot, and follow with the right foot until the feet are hip-width apart again (see figures *b* and *c*). This is 1 rep. Perform all of the reps in one direction; then step to the right to perform all of the reps in that direction.
- Once the prescribed number of X-band walk reps are complete, untwist the band and loop it behind your head and across your shoulders (see figure *d*).
- Initiate the good morning by hinging at the hips and pushing your hips back (see figure *e*).
- Arch the lower back and tuck the chin. Your knees are not locked but also do not move.
- Hinge until you feel the stretch in your hamstrings; then reverse the movement and squeeze the glutes at the top. Perform all reps of the good morning. You have completed 1 set.
- Rest; then perform the next set of X-band walks and good mornings.

Protocol

Sets: 3

Reps: 5 left walks + 5 right walks + 5 good mornings

Rest: 60 sec

Variation

X-Band Walk + Banded Good Morning as a High-Volume Finisher

To perform the X-band walk + banded good morning as a high-volume finisher, follow the same mechanics as described previously, but the amount of resistance will change. In this case, use a moderate to heavy band (0.5-inch [13 mm] thickness); the band thickness should challenge you to perform the recommended 5 reps for each position without stopping.

Protocol

Sets: Max sets in 5 min

Reps: 5 left walks + 5 right walks + 5 good mornings

Rest: As little as possible

In conclusion, isolation exercises should make up a fair amount of any great program. In fact, some would argue isolation exercises should make up the bulk of one's training; however, this will certainly differ on a case-by-case basis. If you have a lower level of experience, you will need to devote more time to improving your foundational patterns. Of course, everyone should work on isolated weaker muscle groups because no one is above training to improve muscular imbalance.

The question becomes, how much time should you devote to specializing in isolation-based exercises? This and more will be fully covered in chapters 9 to 12, where you begin to see that specialization and emphasis on improving limitations increases with your level of experience. Even once you've gained mastery of the foundational patterns, you should still continue to look for where the weak links in the chain present themselves. By doing this you can expect to make constant improvements in maximal strength and body composition. If you're reading this book, it's safe to assume you're not training to get injured, so an emphasis on quality over quantity and identifying weak muscle groups is an appropriate direction to take.

Chapter 8

Plyometric Exercises

Plyometrics are a training tool often associated with athletic development, but their application spans beyond just the field of athletics. As you age, your fast-twitch type II muscle fibers deteriorate, and one way to slow this process is by including plyometric training in your programming on a weekly basis. The good news is that a little bit of plyometric training goes a long way, so you won't need to devote entire training sessions to it. Before we discuss plyometric physiology, let's explore what actually constitutes plyometric training. The easiest and most effective method of plyometric training comes by way of quick, explosive bursts in the form of jumping and landing, bounding, or even a light medicine ball toss. For the sake of simplicity and logistics, we will focus on jumping variations in this chapter. These are the benefits of plyometrics and movements of this type:

- Increased force and power output
- Increased rate of force applied
- Decreased risk of injury in daily activities and athletics
- Increased neural efficiency and coordination
- Increased strength of tendons

Plyometrics take advantage of the stretch-shortening cycle of skeletal muscle, in which a muscle is rapidly lengthened (eccentric contraction) and then voluntarily shortened (concentric contraction). In this cycle, muscles will exhibit an increase in energy (much as when an elastic band is stretched) to produce more power. When programming plyometric exercises, it is important to consider the major impact eccentric contractions have on delayed onset muscle soreness. Eccentric contractions generate about 20 to 60 percent more force than do concentric contractions, leading to an increase in microtrauma (small tearing) of both muscle fibers and connective tissue. Within muscle fibers are muscle spindles that when stretched (during the countermovement portion of the exercise) will send a signal to your central nervous system (CNS) to rapidly contract the lengthened muscle to prevent an overstretch. The faster the rate of stretch, the stronger the signal from the CNS telling that same muscle to contract (known as the stretch reflex) (Potach and Chu 2016).

There are three models of plyometrics that, in essence, capture the key characteristics of not only why plyometrics are so effective, but how plyometrics actually play out physiologically and how positive adaptations can occur when they are programmed correctly (plyometrics programming will be employed in part III of this book). To fully understand plyometrics, you certainly don't need to memorize these models, but understanding the key tenets of each model allows you to better understand the working mechanisms and how plyometric programming can be nuanced (i.e., adding subtle variations to exercises can enhance different aspects of these models such as the storage of elastic energy). The three plyometric models are:

- *Mechanical.* Involves the series elastic component (SEC), the musculotendinous unit that is stretched during eccentric range of motion (ROM). When this occurs, the SEC acts like a lengthened spring and stores elastic energy. It is then able to contribute to total force production by allowing muscles to return to their unstretched configuration.
- *Neurophysiological.* Involves potentiation by way of the stretch reflex, the body's involuntary response to muscles being stretched. The reflexive aspect of plyometrics takes place in muscle spindles.
- *Stretch-shortening.* Employs the energy storage of the SEC and the stimulation of the stretch reflex to facilitate a maximal increase in muscle recruitment.

Now that we understand the basic physiology of plyometric training, let's examine how to use it as part of your training. As mentioned before, fast-twitch type II muscle fiber deteriorates as we age. This is the muscle fiber responsible for gaining lean muscle mass and also has other benefits as it relates to your basal metabolic rate (the rate at which you burn calories at rest). Plyometric work is relatively easy to learn and, depending on the variation you choose, often easy to recover from; it won't take a huge investment of time to learn or to use.

Many strength and conditioning coaches encourage their athletes to use the Olympic lifts to develop explosive strength, but they are not the best choice for speed strength work. Additionally, if you take into consideration the time it takes to learn the Olympic lifts and the number of people who can perform them efficiently enough to derive a speed strength adaptation, there is even less of a case for their inclusion in your program design. When used correctly, plyometric training has been shown to improve the production of muscle force and power, so not only will regular plyometric work help with your overall body composition goal, but it will also improve performance (Potach and Chu 2016). And the feedback I've received after working with thousands of clients has been overwhelmingly positive. Plyometrics will help to keep you engaged in the process of continuous improvement.

Programming Considerations for Plyometrics

Here are a few considerations when designing a training program with plyometrics. It's important to remember that a little bit goes a long way with regard to proper volume distribution of plyometrics.

- *Training age.* A beginner can make the most out of simply learning motor control with jumping and landing and likely does not have to go too far up the hierarchy of plyometric variations provided in this chapter. Adding complexity does not always equate to better results, and the reality is that it can have the opposite effect. Prescribing the best plyometric variation that aligns with the individual is a critical piece of the puzzle.

- *Injury history.* If you have a history of knee and ankle issues, then plyometrics may exacerbate these conditions. This does not mean explosive strength work is out of the question; just use less-demanding variations. This may mean opting for variations that are outside the scope of standard plyometric programming. The usage of other tools like isometrics may be a good alternative.

- *Goals.* If your goals are modest (i.e., improve body composition or longevity), you will likely not need higher-difficulty plyometric variations. On the other hand, if you're a competitive powerlifter, increasing the difficulty of your plyometrics is akin to progressive overload with the squat, bench press, and deadlift. However, as previously stated, higher levels of complexity may not be needed and sometimes regression is the key to sparking new progress.

Also, plyometrics can be used in more than one scenario to provide you with optimal training effects. For example, using plyometrics in the warm-up sequence takes advantage of post-activation potentiation and can prime the sympathetic nervous system for upcoming training; however, the dose needs to align with the desired result. With this in mind, it's important to note that the selected modalities of plyometrics to prime the nervous system for upcoming training will be nearly the same as those to simply develop explosive abilities. (This will be fully covered in the upcoming pages.) The major difference lies with the volume prescriptions. The following table provides the volume prescriptions of plyometric training I've found to be most useful for warm-ups and for training sessions.

Sample exercise	Sets	Reps	Rest
Depth jump at the end of a warm-up sequence	5	3	45 sec
Seated dynamic box jump as main movement in a training session	8	3	60 sec

The goal of using plyometrics in a warm-up is to quickly and effectively prime the CNS prior to training. To accomplish that, no more than 15 total reps (5 sets of 3 reps each) are needed. On the other hand, in a training setting with variations requiring higher levels of skill, about 25 total reps is appropriate.

SEATED DYNAMIC VERTICAL JUMP

This exercise helps you learn how to go from a seated position to a jump to a landing—all of which are critical aspects in safely and effectively performing plyometrics. The dynamic nature of seated-position plyometrics engages the stretch reflex. Learning how to absorb force (in this case through the landing) is important for performing plyometric exercises safely.

Instructions

- Sit on a standard 16-inch (40 cm) weight bench (see figure *a*).
- Keeping the knees bent, lift your feet 4 to 6 inches (10 to 15 cm) off the floor, rocking back on the bench (see figure *b*).
- Bring the feet forcefully back to the ground with the knees bent to initiate your jump while using your arms to initiate forward momentum (see figure *c*).
- Push off the floor with your feet to jump into the air, swinging your arms overhead as you jump up (see figure *d*).
- Land in a partial squat with the hips back and chest up, arms by your sides.
- Immediately sit back down to perform the next jump; repeat until you've completed all repetitions.

Protocol
Sets: 5
Reps: 3
Rest: 45-60 sec

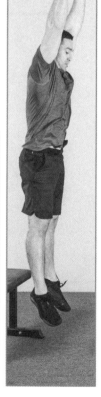

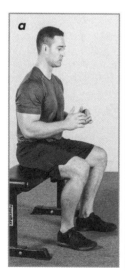
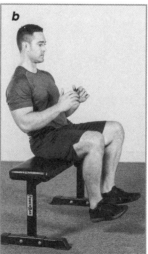
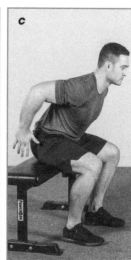

Variation

Seated Dynamic Vertical Jump With Weighted Vest

To perform the seated dynamic vertical jump with weighted vest, use the same mechanics as previously described while adding additional resistance as needed in the form of a weighted vest. All that is needed for added resistance is 10 to 20 pounds (5 to 9 kg) of additional weight. Any more than that may put you at risk of compromising your jump mechanics.

Protocol

Sets: 5

Reps: 3

Rest: 45-60 sec

SEATED DYNAMIC BOX JUMP

This exercise includes aspects similar to the seated dynamic vertical jump but also includes taking the next step of jumping up onto a box, which increases not only the difficulty but the need to use maximal explosion on each repetition. You go dynamically from a seated to a jumping position, culminating with landing and standing on a box.

Instructions

- Sit on a standard 16-inch (40 cm) weight bench (see figure *a*).
- Keeping the knees bent, lift your feet 4 to 6 inches (10 to 15 cm) off the floor, rocking back on the bench (see figure *b*).
- Bring the feet forcefully back to the ground with the knees bent to initiate your jump while using your arms to initiate forward momentum (see figure *c*).
- Push off the floor with your feet to jump into the air, swinging your arms overhead as you jump up (see figure *d*).
- Land on top of the box in a partial squat with the hips back and chest up, arms by your sides (see figure *e*).
- To return to the start position, carefully lower yourself off of the box using your hands for assistance as needed. Avoid jumping off of the top of the box because this could cause injury to the soft tissue of the calves and ankles.
- Immediately perform the next jump until you've completed all repetitions.

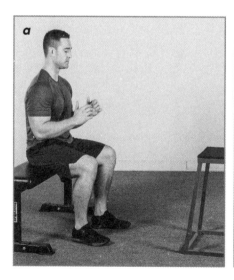
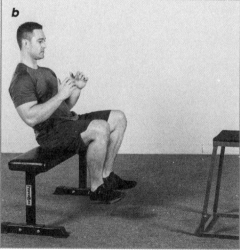

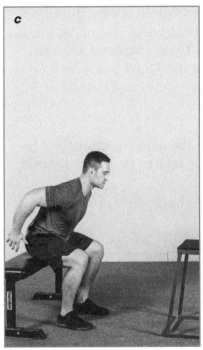
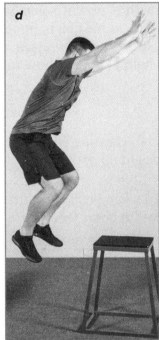
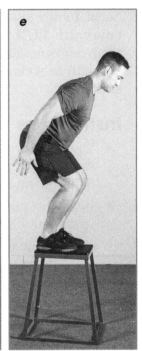

Protocol

Sets: 5

Reps: 3

Rest: 45-60 sec

Variation

Seated Dynamic Box Jump With Weighted Vest

To perform the seated dynamic box jump with weighted vest, use the same mechanics as previously described while adding additional resistance as needed in the form of a weighted vest. The same recommendations regarding weighted vest size apply here—10 to 20 pounds (5 to 9 kg) of additional weight is all that is needed. Any more than that may put you at risk of compromising your jump mechanics.

Protocol

Sets: 5

Reps: 3

Rest: 45-60 sec

Squat jumps start with a partial squat and explosively go through a concentric ROM to a maximal height jump. Both variations of the squat jump shown here are great exercises that will improve explosive strength as well as help you learn how to properly jump and land (absorb force).

Instructions

- Your arms will be assisting each rep in the same manner they assisted in previous jump exercises—using an aggressive arm action to create momentum.
- Begin in a partial squat position with hips back slightly, knees bent, feet about hip-width apart (see figure *a*).
- Jump explosively to a maximal height jump (see figure *b*).
- As you come down, lower into a partial squat to absorb the landing.

Protocol

Sets: 5

Reps: 4

Rest: 45-60 sec

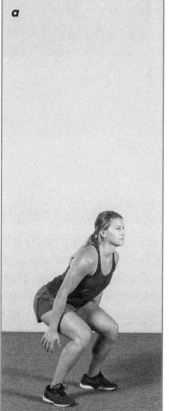
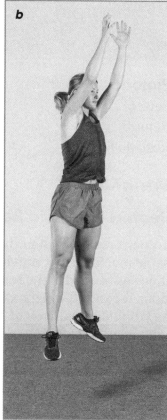

Variation

Band-Assisted Squat Jump

To perform the band-assisted squat jump, affix a heavy-resistance band to a fixed object overhead, preferably a pull-up bar, and use the same mechanics as described previously (see figures *a* and *b*). You'll be using the band to accentuate the ROM on each repetition, but let it be clear that this variation is not for beginners! You should be fully capable of safely landing and initiating each subsequent repetition before attempting the band-assisted variation.

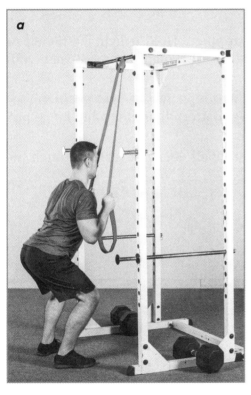
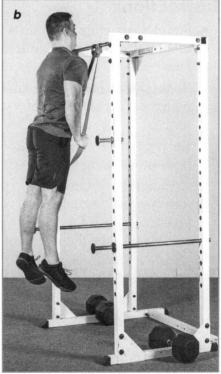

Protocol

Sets: 5
Reps: 4
Rest: 45-60 sec

In the kettlebell squat jump, you hold the kettlebell so that it hangs between your legs as added resistance. The kettlebell does not have to touch the floor upon each repetition, though, as maintaining a neutral spine takes precedence. Loading does not need to be particularly high with this exercise—small loads (35 pounds [16 kg] or less) will go a long way. Also, you must be fully competent with both the hip hinge pattern and the squat pattern before attempting this exercise, since the movement represents a combination of both patterns. If you do not have access to kettlebells, this variation can be performed with a dumbbell.

Instructions

- Stand with your feet hip-width apart. Hold a light kettlebell or dumbbell with both hands, letting the weight hang between your legs.
- Begin by lowering your knees and hips into a squat position (see figure *a*). This is more of a squat pattern than it is a hip hinge pattern.
- Keep your chest lifted. The kettlebell does not have to touch the floor on each rep.
- Explosively jump up, keeping the kettlebell in position, going for maximal height (see figure *b*).
- As you come down, lower into a partial squat to absorb the landing.

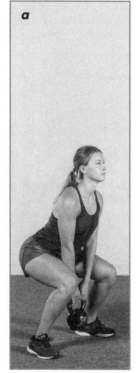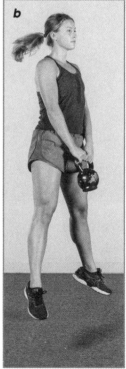

Protocol
Sets: 4
Reps: 4
Rest: 45-60 sec

Variation

Landmine Squat Jump

A squat jump can also be performed with a landmine attachment using light loads. Hold the end of the barbell between your legs with both hands with fingers interlaced. Your hands will stay in this position throughout the entirety of the set (see figures *a* and *b*).

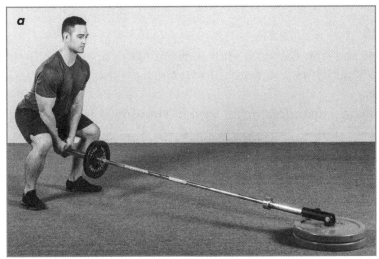

Protocol

Sets: 4

Reps: 4

Rest: 45-60 sec

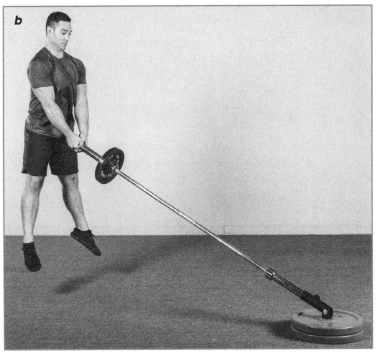

TRAP BAR JUMP

The trap bar adds loading capacity much like the kettlebell but also requires more technical proficiency than other variations. To perform this exercise effectively, you need to be fully competent in the use of the trap bar and the hip hinge pattern. Moreover, even though loading capability is higher with this exercise, heavy loads are not necessary; maximal height of each repetition is the goal. This exercise can be progressed or regressed by simply altering the loading to match your needs.

Instructions

- Stand inside the trap bar with your feet hip-width apart, and bend your knees slightly as you reach down to grasp the handles with both hands.
- Hinge at the hips, maintaining an arch in your lower back (see figure *a*).
- Explosively jump up, extending the hips and keeping the arms straight (see figure *b*).
- As you come down, lower into a partial squat to absorb the landing and lower the empty bar to mid shin position.
- Reset before the next repetition.
- Touch the weight plates to the floor between repetitions.

Protocol

Sets: 5

Reps: 4 @ 20%-30% of deadlift 1RM

Rest: 60 sec

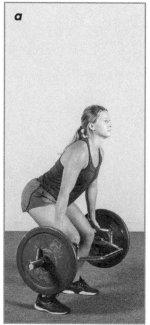 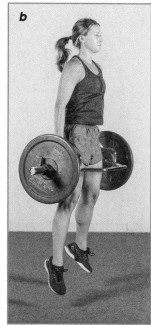

Variation

Beginner Trap Bar Jump

To perform the trap bar jump when learning the technique, use the same mechanics as described previously, but use the trap bar without any weight plates. You will not touch the trap bar to the floor between repetitions.

Protocol

Sets: 3

Reps: 3

Rest: 60 sec

The barbell squat jump is an excellent variation that emphasizes the squat pattern with the barbell placed in the back rack position. Like the trap bar, the barbell has a high loading capacity, but jumping with it also requires more technical proficiency with the squat pattern and the ability to effectively absorb force with added resistance. (The kettlebell squat jump is a great regression to this and should be mastered before progressing to this variation.) To be clear, this variation is *not* performed with a full squat on each rep—stay above parallel to make this a more rapid movement. This exercise can be progressed or regressed by simply altering the loading to match your needs.

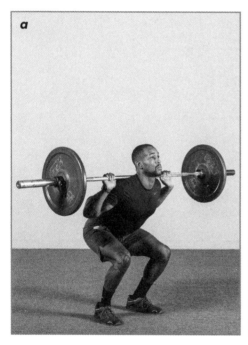
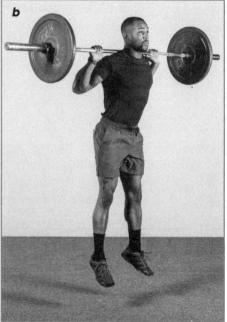

Instructions

- Start with the barbell in the back rack position (barbell placed on your mid traps) with feet hip-width apart.
- Lower into a partial squat position by bending your knees and pushing your hips back (see figure *a*).
- Jump explosively to a maximal height jump by extending the hips and knees, keeping the barbell in place (see figure *b*).
- As you come down, lower into a partial squat to absorb your landing; then initiate your next repetition.

Protocol

Sets: 5

Reps: 4 @ 20%-30% of back squat 1RM

Rest: 60 sec

Variation

Beginner Barbell Squat Jump

To perform the barbell squat jump when learning the technique, use the same mechanics as described previously, but use a barbell without any weight plates.

Protocol

Sets: 3

Reps: 3

Rest: 60 sec

SINGLE-LEG BOX JUMP

The single-leg box jump adds to the technical proficiency required for jumping and landing. The jump is performed unilaterally, which will force you to refine your jumping and landing mechanics to a lower box height. This variation is not for beginners or for general fitness training but can be a great option for athletes who engage in explosive sports like American football.

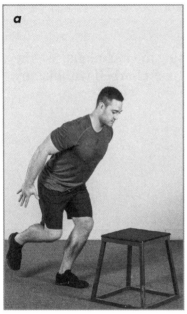
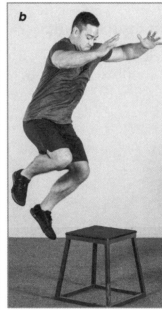
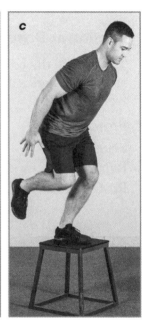

Instructions

- Stand facing a low box, around 16 to 20 inches (40 to 50 cm) in height, in a partial squat with feet hip-width apart, knees slightly bent, hips pushed back, arms by your sides.
- Pick one foot up and prepare to jump with the leg you're standing on (see figure *a*).
- Use your arms to help you explosively jump up as you propel yourself forward and up onto the box, landing on the jumping leg (see figures *b* and *c*).
- Jump back down on both legs, lowering into the partial squat position to absorb the landing. This is 1 rep.
- Complete the reps on one leg; then switch legs.

Protocol

Sets: 6
Reps: 2 each side
Rest: 45-60 sec

Variation

Half-Kneeling Single-Leg Box Jump

To progress, perform the half-kneeling single-leg box jump by using the same mechanics as described previously, but from a half-kneeling position (see figures *a-c*). This variation requires a great deal of coordination, balance, and accuracy.

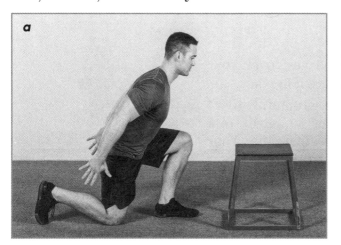

Protocol

Sets: 6

Reps: 2 each side

Rest: 45-60 sec

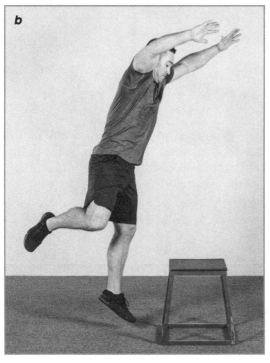

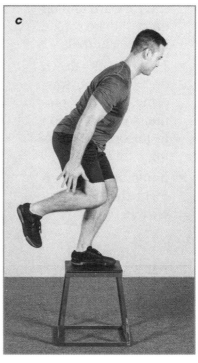

WEIGHTED BOX JUMP

As we progress plyometric variations, increasing resistance would seem to make sense, but this isn't always the case. With the weighted box jump, either seated or standing, we add load in the form of dumbbells or weighted vests, but a little goes a long way (e.g., 10- to 20-pound [5 to 9 kg] dumbbells or a 10- to 20-pound [5 to 9 kg] weighted vest). The addition of load should not compromise jumping and landing techniques. Weighted box jumps are done optimally with a weighted vest, which leaves you the use of your hands if by chance you slip up.

Instructions

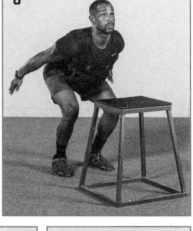

- Place the weighted vest over your shoulders and secure it in place.
- Stand facing a box around 20 to 24 inches (50 to 60 cm) in height, in a partial squat (see figure *a*). Your feet should be hip-width apart, your knees slightly bent, your hips pushed back, and your arms by your sides.
- Use your arms to help you explosively jump up as you propel yourself forward and up onto the box (see figures *b* and *c*).
- Jump back down on both legs, lowering into the partial squat position to absorb the landing.
- Immediately perform the next repetition.

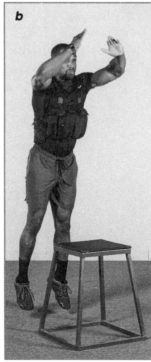

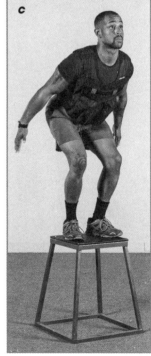

Protocol
Sets: 8
Reps: 2
Rest: 60 sec

Variation

Dumbbell Box Jump

To perform the dumbbell box jump, use the same mechanics as described previously, but hold a dumbbell in each hand, keeping your arms by your sides as you jump (see figures *a-c*). With regard to loading, start with 10 to 20 pounds (5 to 9 kg) and get comfortable before adding any more weight. You'll likely find not much more is needed beyond that; the goal is always to maximize training effects without increasing the risk of injury.

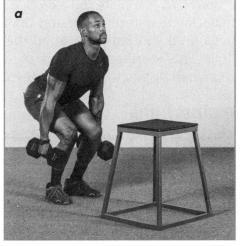

Protocol

Sets: 8

Reps: 2

Rest: 60 sec

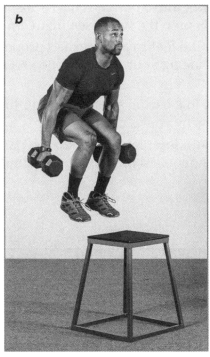

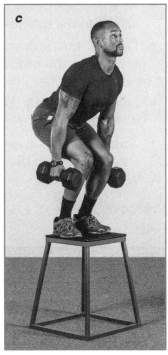

DUMBBELL SQUAT JUMP + BOX JUMP

The dumbbell squat jump + box jump combines the dumbbell squat jump and a box jump as one powerful unit. Because you are starting the movement with added resistance and then using a jettison technique to release the dumbbells before going into your box jump, you are effectively utilizing post-activation potentiation. To perform this exercise correctly, you should be fully competent and able to perform a trap bar jump (page 172); this is a progression to that exercise due to the position of the dumbbells in relation to the body and the mechanics required to complete the exercise safely and effectively. This exercise takes some coordination and timing, so practice first without dumbbells until you have mastered the motions, and then add the dumbbells. This exercise can be progressed by adding dumbbell loading and regressed by simply not using the dumbbells.

Instructions

- Stand facing a box, around 20 to 24 inches (50 to 60 cm) in height, in a partial squat (see figure *a*). Your feet should be hip-width apart, your knees slightly bent, your hips pushed back, and your arms by your sides. Hold a dumbbell in each hand.
- Jump explosively to a maximal height jump, keeping the arms straight and dumbbells at your sides (see figure *b*).
- As you come down, lower into a partial squat to absorb the landing and drop the dumbbells onto the floor (see figure *c*).
- Push off the floor with the feet to jump up and propel yourself forward onto the box, swinging your arms overhead as you jump up (see figure *d*).
- Land on top of the box in a partial squat with your hips back, your chest up, and your arms by your sides (see figure *e*).
- Jump back down on both legs, lowering into the partial squat position to absorb the landing and picking up the dumbbells for the next repetition.

Protocol
Sets: 5
Reps: 2 (1 dumbbell squat jump + 1 box jump)
Rest: 60 sec

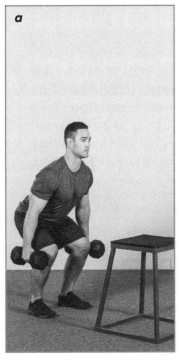

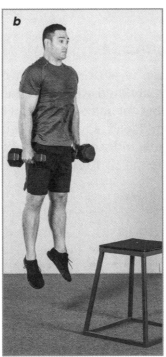

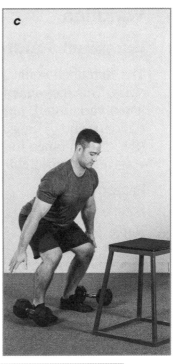

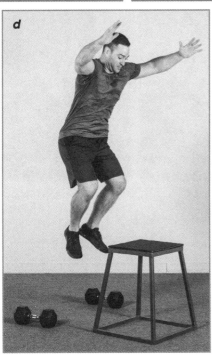

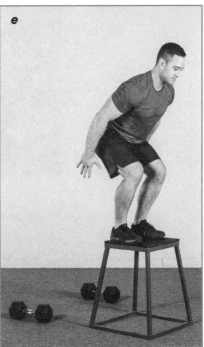

Variation

Dumbbell Squat Jump

The dumbbell squat jump is performed with dumbbells held by your sides. This movement is initiated with a partial squat (much like other listed variations), jumping for maximal height on each repetition (see figures *a* and *b*). Suggested load is relatively light, in the 20- to 30-pound (9 to 14 kg) range for most individuals will suffice, but that's not to say you cannot start lighter in the 10- to 20-pound (5 to 9 kg) range if needed.

Protocol

Sets: 5
Reps: 3
Rest: 45-60 sec

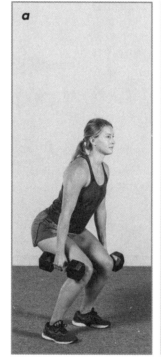
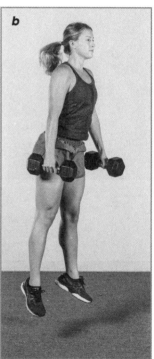

LATERAL BOX JUMP

The lateral box jump is a great way to train movement in the frontal plane, which is critical to athletic performance. It's recommended to start with a box height lower than that for the traditional standing box jump because the movement is not as familiar for most athletes. A standard bench height of 16 inches (40 cm) will work well before advancing to a higher level. This movement requires a fair amount of coordination and certainly isn't for beginners. You'll be performing this exercise explosively with no pauses between reps.

Instructions

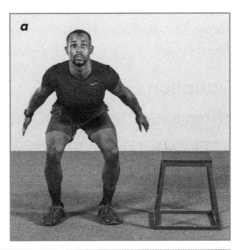

- Stand with your left side to a bench or 16-inch (40 cm) box, in a partial squat (see figure *a*). Your feet should be hip-width apart, your knees slightly bent, your hips pushed back, and your arms by your sides.
- Use your arms to help you explosively jump up laterally as you propel yourself to your

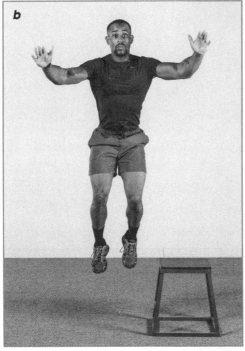

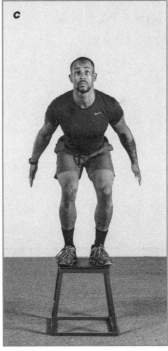

left (think of a ski jump motion) and up onto the box (see figures *b* and *c*).

- Jump back down to the floor, lowering into a partial squat position to absorb the landing, and immediately initiate your next repetition.
- After completing the repetitions on the left side, switch to the right.

Protocol

Sets: 6
Reps: 2 each side
Rest: 60 sec

Variation

Lateral Box Jump With Weighted Vest

To progress, perform the lateral box jump with weighted vest, using the same mechanics as described previously, but while wearing a 10- to 20-pound (5 to 9 kg) load in a weighted vest. Anything higher than that is not recommended because it will add undue stress to soft tissue.

Protocol

Sets: 5
Reps: 2 each side
Rest: 60 sec

DEPTH JUMP

While the depth jump is a viable option for explosive strength work, it is often done incorrectly. There are a few caveats to adding the depth jump to your training program. First, resist the urge to go higher than a 20-inch (50 cm) box because absorbing the landing from any higher can present risk to soft tissue. Second, because of the accelerated eccentric phase of this movement, adding additional resistance is not necessary.

Instructions

- Stand on top of a standard 16-inch (40 cm) bench or box with your feet about hip-width apart and your toes near the edge.
- Let one foot hover in front of you, off the box, to start the movement (see figure *a*).
- Step off the bench, landing in a partial squat with your arms extended behind you in an athletic position (see figure *b*).
- Turn around to step back onto the box for the next repetition.
- Complete the reps on one leg; then switch legs.

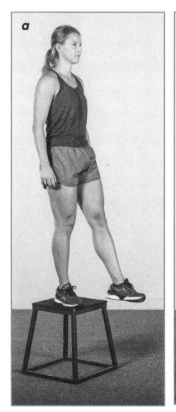

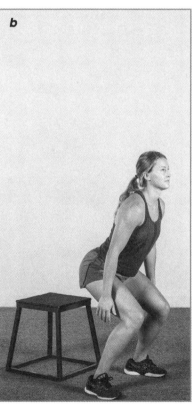

Protocol

Sets: 5

Reps: 2 each side

Rest: 60 sec

Variation

Depth Jump + Vertical Jump

To progress, perform the depth jump in conjunction with other plyometric variations such as a vertical jump, using the same mechanics for the depth jump as described previously. Immediately after you land in an athletic position with your arms behind you, you'll swing your arms forward and upward as you initiate your vertical jump for maximal height (see figures *a-c*); then land again in that same athletic position to end the movement.

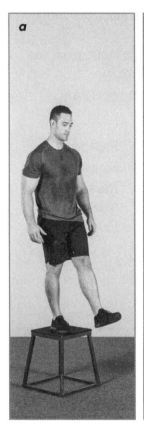
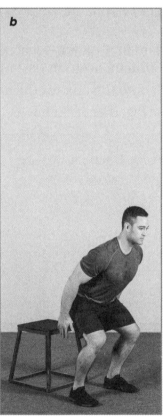
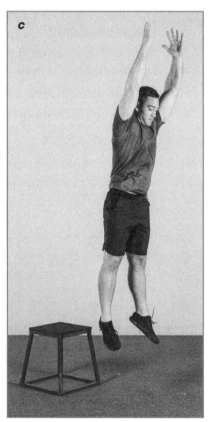

Protocol

Sets: 5
Reps: 1 depth jump + 1 vertical jump each side
Rest: 60 sec

KNEELING JUMP

The kneeling jump is an advanced exercise bringing you dynamically from a kneeling position to a partial squat to a standing position. This is not a variation for beginners because the level of motor control and explosive ability required is quite high. This exercise can be performed with either a dynamic or a static start, the latter being less difficult than the former.

Instructions

- Start from a kneeling position with your chest held high and your arms by your sides (see figure *a*).
- Bring your hips back to your heels to start the dynamic portion of this exercise (see figure *b*).
- Move explosively through hip extension, bringing your knees off the floor and jumping into a parallel squat (quarter squat if possible) with the feet hip-width apart (see figures *c* and *d*). You can swing your arms during the jump.
- Fully stand up, and return to the kneeling position to start the next repetition.

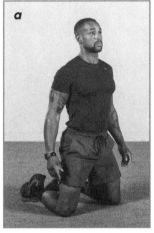
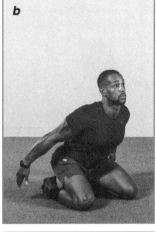
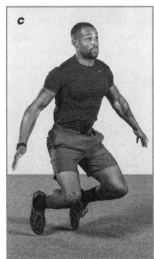
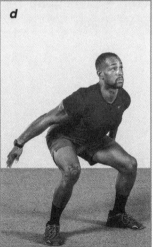

Protocol

Sets: 6
Reps: 3
Rest: 60 sec

Variation

Kneeling Jump + Box Jump

To progress, perform the kneeling jump in conjunction with other plyometric variations such as a box jump, which increases the demand on your explosive ability. Use the same mechanics as described previously, adding the secondary movement of jumping onto the box. After initiating the kneeling jump, go explosively right into your box jump using your arms to help propel you forward and upward (see figures *a-d*). For advanced athletes, this variation can be performed with a weighted vest of 10 to 20 pounds (5 to 9 kg).

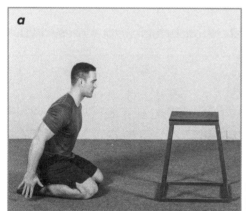

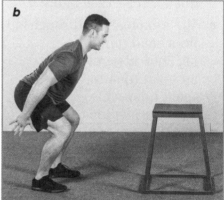

Protocol
Sets: 8
Reps: 1 kneeling jump + 1 box jump
Rest: 60 sec

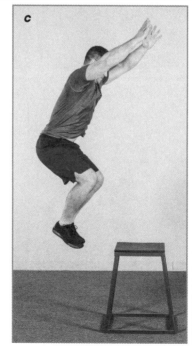

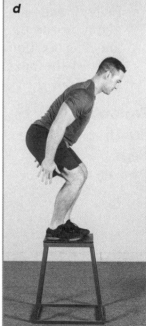

In conclusion, plyometrics are an aspect of training typically more prevalent in athletics. However, now that you understand the physiology, you can see that it makes sense to invest at least a minimal amount of time in plyometric training. The training is safe and effective, and can be tailored to your personal needs, goals, and training age.

PART III

THE PROGRAMS

Chapter 9

Hypertrophy Programs

Hypertrophy work, accessory work, special exercise work, single-joint work, unilateral work—whatever you'd like to call it, it's a staple in any great training program. For some individuals, performing hypertrophy work alone as the crux of their training plan is prudent. Hypertrophy work is beneficial from a number of perspectives and can span all abilities, so whether you're a seasoned lifter or a newbie, hypertrophy work will be an integral part of your training plan. Moreover, hypertrophy work can act as a primer for strength development while encouraging better motor-unit synchronization, symmetry, and resilience. Furthermore, hypertrophy work is a great way to add lean tissue in the beginning stages of one's training. But I'd be remiss if I didn't lay out why a hypertrophy-based training plan is effective for a wide array of individuals looking to improve numerous aspects of their training.

BENEFITS OF HYPERTROPHY WORK

Because hypertrophy-style training programs are an important form of training, particularly for individuals with low training ages, let's discuss some of the benefits this work can have, as well as its carryover to other aspects of fitness.

- *Potential to increase calorie expenditure.* Even though the increase in metabolic rate is not as large as we once thought it was, hypertrophy work can be a factor in caloric expenditure, fat loss, and blood sugar regulation when you add a significant amount of lean mass.
- *High amounts of time under tension.* Just as a bodybuilder spends a significant amount of time isolating specific muscle groups, we

can employ a high volume of hypertrophy work. In an effort to target where we may be lacking, we can add a high volume of work without the risk of exacerbating faulty motor patterns. This work allows athletes of all levels to perform work without being limited by their lack of skill; because it's low skill, just about everyone can derive benefits.

- *Reduced risk versus reward.* It is safer to add volume to single-joint movements than to multijoint movements, just as it's safer to increase the volume of a unilateral movement like a split squat than the volume of a bilateral movement like a back squat. Additionally, increasing the volume on compound movements carries a higher risk of overuse injury, which could hinder success even though you worked hard in a training session.

- *Reduced neural demand.* Building on our last benefit, unilateral work requires less skill and neural demand, so we can increase loading and volume commensurately, thereby increasing the time under tension. This leads to an increase in muscular hypertrophy. Most who believe assistance exercises are unnecessary are simply uninformed about their influence on body composition. With lower neural demand comes less potential of central fatigue and thus lower risk of overtraining.

- *Increased potential to generate force.* Just about any exercise physiology book or study will confirm this. While you may not see performing direct biceps work carry over to your pull-ups right away, you'll see substantial improvements in as little as eight weeks (Haff 2016).

- *Improved performance of multijoint movements.* If you want to make improvements when performing movements like squats, deadlifts, and Olympic lifts, it makes sense to prioritize training where you are weakest. Single-joint movements and isolation exercises allow you to add more direct posterior chain work to address weaknesses in all of these lifts.

- *Reduced risk of injury.* You can effectively reduce the risk of injury as well as rehabilitate current injuries with hypertrophy work. It's critical to constantly assess where you are most limited and take inventory of nagging aches and pains. For example, lower back disorder injuries are rising at an alarming rate, making direct gluteal and hip work a great place to focus hypertrophy efforts.

Hypertrophy work has the power to help individuals reach their full potential, and performing this work alone can help one reset and reprogram faulty motor patterns as well as add lean muscle mass. Moreover, for individuals who are still learning how to move and perform patterns like the squat and the hip hinge, exercises with less overall complexity and risk of technical error (think of a split squat versus a back squat) are a great place to start to improve motor control and facilitate long-term training sustainability.

HYPERTROPHY PROGRAMS

First, let's discuss the ideal training splits for using these programs. While this book focuses on strategies for the lower body, knowing where to place these training days within the training cycle is important so that you're including upper body–centric days as well as conditioning days (the type of training on these days is called energy systems development, or ESD). To help you do that effectively, table 9.1 shows five training split options to ensure that proper nervous system recovery is built in. Recommended conditioning work (ESD) is included in these splits as well. (It's highly recommended that you include ESD in your training.) Total-body training is also included, which is a form of training that aims to train both lower body and upper body modalities in one session.

This chapter includes four blocks of beginner-intermediate programming and four blocks of advanced programming. Despite this separation into beginner-intermediate and advanced programs, the connection between all three levels of programming is stronger than you might think because the primary goal across all levels is to train foundational movement patterns. The difference between beginner, intermediate, and advanced lies in the complexity of exercise variations, the choice in training methods (i.e., maximal effort versus submaximal effort), and the level of volume prescribed.

Table 9.1 Sample Training Split Options for Hypertrophy Training

	Day 1	Day 2	Day 3	Day 4	Day 5	Day 6	Day 7
Training split option 1	Lower	ESD	Upper	ESD	Lower	Upper	OFF
Training split option 2	Upper	Lower	ESD	Upper	Lower	ESD	OFF
Training split option 3	Upper	ESD	Lower	ESD	Upper	ESD	Lower
Training split option 4	Lower	ESD	Upper	ESD	Total	OFF	OFF
Training split option 5	Total	ESD	Total	ESD	Total	ESD	OFF

BEGINNER-INTERMEDIATE PROGRAM
WITH HYPERTROPHY EMPHASIS

BLOCK 1

Program Notes

- This training split can be run for 3 to 4 weeks.
- Increase training volume as your movement quality improves.
- Emphasize ingraining good motor patterns versus volume or load.
- This session should be separated from your other lower body sessions by 72 hours.

Exercise	Page	Sets	Reps	Rest
1. Single-leg landmine Romanian deadlift	103	3-4	6-8 each side	90 sec
2. Goblet box squat	75	3-4	10-12	60 sec
3. Barbell banded glute hip thrust	152	3-4	12-15	60 sec
4. Dumbbell split squat	53	3-4	8-10 each side	60 sec
5. Single-leg dumbbell calf raise	131	3-4	8-10 each side	60 sec

Program Notes

- This training split can be run for 3 to 4 weeks.
- Increase training volume as your movement quality improves.
- Emphasize ingraining good motor patterns versus volume or load.
- This session should be separated from your other lower body sessions by 72 hours.

Exercise		Page	Sets	Reps	Rest
1. Trap bar deadlift		116	5	Build to a heavy 5 or 5RM	2-3 min
2. Goblet box squat		75	3-4	10-12	60 sec
3. Glute-ham raise		112	3-4	6-8	90 sec
4. Landmine lateral squat		72	3-4	6-8 each side	90 sec
5. Cable pull-through		94	3-4	15-20	60 sec

BEGINNER-INTERMEDIATE PROGRAM
WITH HYPERTROPHY EMPHASIS *(continued)*

BLOCK 3

Program Notes
- This training split can be run for 3 to 4 weeks.
- Increase training volume as your movement quality improves.
- Emphasize ingraining good motor patterns versus volume or load.
- This session should be separated from your other lower body sessions by 72 hours.

Exercise		Page	Sets	Reps	Rest
1. Trap bar deadlift		116	5	Build to a heavy 5 or 5RM	2-3 min
2. Glute-ham raise		112	3-4	6-8	90 sec
3. 1-1/4 dumbbell split squat		54	2-3	12-15 each side (1 full ROM rep + 1/4 rep at the bottom of each rep = 1 rep)	45-60 sec
4. Band-resisted glute bridge		142	3	8-10	60 sec
5. Backward sled drag (heavy load)		51	6	30 yd (27 m)	60-90 sec

Program Notes

- This training split can be run for 3 to 4 weeks.
- The last two exercises are performed as a superset, going back and forth between both until all sets are complete.
- Increase training volume as your movement quality improves.
- Emphasize ingraining good motor patterns versus volume or load.
- This session should be separated from your other lower body sessions by 72 hours.

Exercise		Page	Sets	Reps	Rest
1. Barbell front box squat		81	5-8	1-5RM	2.5 min
2. Barbell glute hip thrust		98	4-5	8-10	90 sec
3. Landmine lateral squat		72	3-4	6-8 each side	90 sec
4. Banded pull-through		154	4	25	60 sec
5. Seated double-leg banded hamstring curl		140	4	25+	60 sec

ADVANCED PROGRAM WITH HYPERTROPHY EMPHASIS

BLOCK 1

Program Notes

- This training split can be run for 3 to 4 weeks.
- Increase training volume as your movement quality improves.
- Emphasize ingraining good motor patterns versus volume or load.
- This session should be separated from your other lower body sessions by 72 hours.

Exercise	Page	Sets	Reps	Rest
1. Sumo stance rack deadlift	120	8	Build to a 1RM	3 min
2. Goblet box squat	75	3-4	10-12	60 sec
3. Barbell glute hip thrust	98	4-5	8-10	90 sec
4. Dumbbell walking lunge	60	3	20 total steps (10 on each leg)	60-90 sec
5. Forward sled drag (heavy load)	91	6-10	60 yd (55 m)	60-90 sec

Program Notes

- This training split can be run for 3 to 4 weeks.
- Increase training volume as your movement quality improves.
- Emphasize ingraining good motor patterns versus volume or load.
- This session should be separated from your other lower body sessions by 72 hours.

Exercise		Page	Sets	Reps	Rest
1. Barbell front box squat		81	5-8	1-5RM	2.5 min
2. Trap bar Romanian deadlift		117	4	8-10	90 sec to 2 min
3. Landmine lateral squat		72	3-4	6-8 each side	90 sec
4. Cable pull-through		94	3-4	15-20	60 sec
5. Backward sled drag (heavy load)		51	6	30 yd (27 m)	60-90 sec

ADVANCED PROGRAM WITH
HYPERTROPHY EMPHASIS *(continued)*

BLOCK 3

Program Notes
- This training split can be run for 3 to 4 weeks.
- Increase training volume as your movement quality improves.
- Emphasize ingraining good motor patterns versus volume or load.
- This session should be separated from your other lower body sessions by 72 hours.

Exercise	Page	Sets	Reps	Rest
1. Sumo stance Romanian deadlift with bands pulling forward	106	4-5	8-10	90 sec to 2 min
2. Rear-foot elevated split squat	63	3-4	6-10 each side	90 sec
3. Medicine ball loaded back raise	101	4	15-20	60 sec
4. Goblet squat	76	3-4	12-15	60 sec
5. Forward sled drag (heavy load)	91	6-10	60 yd (55 m)	60-90 sec

Program Notes

- This training split can be run for 3 to 4 weeks.
- For the barbell front box squat clusters, build to a heavy 6 (a load that is heavy for 6 reps but not necessarily a 6RM) and rest for 2 minutes between sets. Then perform 3 cluster sets of 3 reps, rerack, and rest for 20 seconds. Next, do 2 reps, rerack, and rest for 20 seconds. Finally, do 1 rep, rerack, and rest for 3 minutes. This should be done at 80 to 85 percent of 1RM front squat.
- Increase training volume as your movement quality improves.
- Emphasize ingraining good motor patterns versus volume or load.
- This session should be separated from your other lower body sessions by 72 hours.

Exercise		Page	Sets	Reps	Rest
1. Barbell front box squat clusters		83	3	3.2.1 (20 sec)	3 min
2. Loaded glute-ham raise (with weighted vest)		115	4	6-8	90 sec
3. Dumbbell walking lunge		60	3	20 total steps (10 on each leg)	60-90 sec
4. Cable pull-through		94	3-4	15-20	60 sec
5. Seated single-leg banded hamstring curl		138	5	25 each side	As needed

In conclusion, hypertrophy-based programs are an excellent starting point for individuals who may not yet be ready to handle bilateral patterns using heavier loads. This work sets the stage for good motor patterns, good motor-unit recruitment, and creating resilience in the skeletal system. Or, if you need a "reset" after time off from the gym, a hypertrophy-based program may be the best place to start before you advance to a strength or athletic performance program.

Chapter 10

Strength Programs

In chapter 3, we covered the physiology of strength training and talked in depth about strength training's benefits as well as how it can help create synergy within a training program. In this chapter, we'll see what those training programs look like and highlight three methods of arriving at strength training adaptations. It's important to note that not all strength training is created equal; a well-rounded training plan will include multiple methods of developing strength. Furthermore, although the programs included in this chapter are geared toward developing strength, you'll still see similarities between these programs and other programs in this book because there is carryover between developing strength, hypertrophy, and athletic performance. The methods put forward in this book are multifaceted and can be used for many purposes. For example, plyometrics can be used for athletic performance and as a tool to slow the aging process for general fitness athletes. It's important to look at the development of one quality on a continuum that encompasses all qualities of strength because one does not develop maximal strength or athletic performance alone and many variables go into accomplishing those goals.

CREATING STRENGTH TRAINING ADAPTATIONS

Developing strength involves more than just lifting heavy loads. The reality is that force comes in many shapes and sizes and while we know by definition strength is the ability of a muscle or muscle group to generate force, having a well-rounded approach to achieving strength gains is a smarter alternative than just lifting heavy. In this chapter, we'll discuss two methods of strength development that will be critical to your success in the gym. We'll discuss why you should consider utilizing these methods along with their benefits, their reasoning, and how they play a part in keeping your programming balanced (in order to avoid things like overtraining). For more information about other training methods, see chapter 3.

Dynamic Effort Training

It's a common misconception that you need to lift heavy in every workout. Many think that the effectiveness of training is judged by how hard it is. But the human body isn't a gumball machine—it doesn't spit out candy every time you put a quarter in. That's because there is a point of diminishing returns. If you're not allowing for proper recovery between higher-threshold, or maximal lifting, sessions (sessions that are more demanding on the central nervous system), you'll eventually overtrain and start losing your progress or get injured. The reality is that hard training sessions need to be interspersed with easier training sessions. It's also important to incorporate strength methods that differ with regard to bar velocity.

What does this mean to the average individual who wants to get stronger? It means that there is low-hanging fruit to be picked with methods such as dynamic effort (DE) training, which aims to improve strength through nonmaximal measures that activate high-threshold motor units to a high degree. The goal of this method is to use nonmaximal loads with the highest attainable velocity (bar speed) to improve the rate of force development (RFD) and increase the number of recruited and trained motor units (Zatsiorsky, Kraemer, and Fry 2021).

These are the key features of DE training:

- Uses high-threshold motor units and facilitates RFD
- Places high demands on the nervous system
- Works best with accommodating resistance (AR) to ensure proper loading throughout full range of motion (ROM). AR is the use of bands or chains to provide maximal tension through full ROM.

- Must be separated from maximal effort training by at least 72 hours
- Works the velocity portion of the force-velocity curve

In short, DE training is used in this book both for strength development and athletic performance. This method maximizes the velocity component of the force-velocity curve while creating balanced programming to reduce the risk of overtraining.

Submaximal Effort Training

The repeated effort method, covered in chapter 3, is an integral aspect of every program in this book. While there are some similarities between it and the submaximal effort method, the major difference is that submaximal work is delivered exclusively through bilateral movements (i.e., squats, presses, pulls). The submaximal effort method will be used as a multiple-repetition maximum scenario (two- to six-rep max) because true maximal effort training consists of a singular one-rep maximal load set.

The goal with the submaximal effort method is twofold: (1) to develop proper motor patterns with bilateral movements approaching heavier loads and (2) to improve strength qualities via recruitment of high-threshold motor units and thus improve neuromuscular efficiency. Furthermore, this method is a prerequisite for maximal effort training, meaning that one should have first developed efficient movement before considering attempting maximal effort lifts. Moreover, the submaximal effort method can be used strategically for autoregulation. Stress affects all individuals differently, and asking someone to adhere to rigid percentages (five sets of three reps at 75 percent of one-rep max) does *not* account for daily fluctuations. Using submaximal effort training allows the individual to build up in weight based on how they are feeling on any given day. This method is also easier to navigate because building to a heavy triple for the day is less confusing than adhering to strict percentage-based guidelines. Submaximal effort training works both aspects of the force-velocity curve while creating balanced programming to reduce the risk of overtraining.

STRENGTH PROGRAMS

First, let's discuss the ideal training splits for using these programs. While this book focuses on strategies for the lower body, knowing where to place these training days within the training cycle is important so that you're including upper body–centric days as well as energy systems development (ESD). In regard to ESD training, while this book isn't intended to go into the nuances of training the aerobic and anaerobic systems, knowing where conditioning fits into a training template is important to ensure your training program is well-rounded. A well-designed program will likely include conditioning, particularly for the aerobic system, which has the ability to improve recoverability between your main strength sessions. Aerobic conditioning does not need to be overly complicated, and you can improve work capacity as well as your ability to recover between sessions by including one to two aerobic sessions per week performing steady-state cyclical work (i.e., Stairmaster, treadmill, air bike, light sled pulls) for 20 to 30 minutes keeping your heart rate at 60 to 70 percent of max heart rate. This will not only help build your aerobic capacity but also improve things like cardiac output, which is your heart's ability to pump blood to your extremities.

If regular conditioning is not a part of your program, I'd still recommend using ESD days as listed in the program to perform modalities like sled work (sled drag variations are mentioned several times throughout this book in both chapters 5 and 6) as a bridge between your main training sessions. Table 10.1 shows five training split options that will allow for proper nervous system recovery between sessions. These splits assume that you use a concurrent approach to training (i.e., training multiple qualities of both strength and conditioning within the same week of training).

This chapter includes four blocks of beginner-intermediate programming and four blocks of advanced programming. Despite this separation into beginner-intermediate and advanced programs, the connection between all three levels of programming is stronger than you might think because the primary goal across all levels is to train foundational movement patterns. The difference between beginner, intermediate, and advanced lies in the complexity of exercise variations, the choice in training methods (i.e., maximal effort versus submaximal effort), and the level of volume prescribed.

Table 10.1 Sample Training Split Options for Strength Training

	Day 1	Day 2	Day 3	Day 4	Day 5	Day 6	Day 7
Training split option 1	Lower	ESD	Upper	ESD	Lower	Upper	OFF
Training split option 2	Upper	Lower	ESD	Upper	Lower	ESD	OFF
Training split option 3	Upper	ESD	Lower	ESD	Upper	ESD	Lower
Training split option 4	Lower	ESD	Upper	ESD	Total	OFF	OFF
Training split option 5	Total	ESD	Total	ESD	Total	ESD	OFF

BEGINNER-INTERMEDIATE PROGRAM WITH STRENGTH EMPHASIS

BLOCK 1

Program Notes

- This training split can be run for 3 to 4 weeks.
- For the trap bar deadlift, build to a heavy 3 to 5 reps in 5 or more sets.
- Increase training volume as your movement quality improves.
- Emphasize ingraining good motor patterns versus volume or load.
- This session should be separated from your other lower body sessions by 72 hours.

Exercise		Page	Sets	Reps	Rest
1. Trap bar deadlift		116	5	Build to a heavy 3-5RM	2-3 min
2. Goblet box squat		75	3-4	10-12	60 sec
3. Barbell banded glute hip thrust		152	3-4	12-15	60 sec
4. Dumbbell split squat		53	2-3	8-10 each side	60 sec
5. X-band walk + banded good morning		156	3	5 left walks + 5 right walks + 5 good mornings	60 sec

Program Notes

- This training split can be run for 3 to 4 weeks.
- For the barbell front box squat, perform 8 sets × 3 reps for speed (dynamic effort using 50 to 60 percent of 1RM back squat to 16-inch [40 cm] box). Each week, add 3 to 5 percent to your load while maintaining bar velocity.
- Increase training volume as your movement quality improves.
- Emphasize ingraining good motor patterns versus volume or load.
- This session should be separated from your other lower body sessions by 72 hours.

Exercise		Page	Sets	Reps	Rest
1. Barbell front box squat		81	5-8	1-5RM	2.5 min
2. Glute-ham raise		112	3-4	6-8	90 sec
3. Goblet squat		76	3-4	12-15	60 sec
4. Cable pull-through		94	3-4	15-20	60 sec
5. Seated calf raise		146	3	12-15	60 sec

BEGINNER-INTERMEDIATE PROGRAM
WITH STRENGTH EMPHASIS *(continued)*

BLOCK 3

Program Notes
- This training split can be run for 3 to 4 weeks.
- For the Anderson front squat, build to 3RM set with pins so you start at parallel. Each week, build to a heavy 4 in week 1; a heavy 3 in week 2; a heavy 2 in week 3; and a heavy 1 in week 4.
- Increase training volume as your movement quality improves.
- Emphasize ingraining good motor patterns versus volume or load.
- This session should be separated from your other lower body sessions by 72 hours.

Exercise	Page	Sets	Reps	Rest
1. Anderson front squat	78	Build in weight over the course of 5 sets	5RM	2.5 min
2. Band-assisted glute-ham raise	114	4	6-8	90 sec
3. Landmine reverse lunge	57	3-4	8-10 each side	60 sec
4. Band-resisted glute bridge	142	3	8-10	60 sec
5. Backward sled drag (moderate load)	51	6	30 yd (27 m)	60-90 sec

Program Notes

- This training split can be run for 3 to 4 weeks.
- For the sumo stance deadlift against a band for dynamic effort, use 60 to 70 percent of 1RM, adding 5 percent each week.
- Increase training volume as your movement quality improves.
- Emphasize ingraining good motor patterns versus volume or load.
- This session should be separated from your other lower body sessions by 72 hours.

Exercise		Page	Sets	Reps	Rest
1. Sumo stance deadlift against a band for dynamic effort		123	6	2 @ 50% of 1RM + band tension	60 sec
2. Barbell front rack reverse lunge		69	5	5 each side	90 sec to 2 min
3. Barbell glute hip thrust		98	4-5	8-10	90 sec
4. Goblet box squat		75	3-4	10-12	60 sec
5. Lateral sled drag (moderate load)		129	6	30 yd (27 m) each side	60-90 sec

ADVANCED PROGRAM WITH STRENGTH EMPHASIS

BLOCK 1

Program Notes

- This training split can be run for 3 to 4 weeks.
- For the trap bar deadlift clusters, perform 3 reps, then rest for 15 seconds; perform 2 reps, then rest for 15 seconds; and finally perform 1 rep, and rest a full 3 minutes.
- Increase training volume as your movement quality improves.
- Emphasize ingraining good motor patterns versus volume or load.
- This session should be separated from your other lower body sessions by 72 hours.

Exercise		Page	Sets	Reps	Rest
1. Trap bar deadlift clusters		119	3	3.2.1 (15 sec)	3 min
2. Goblet squat		76	3-4	8-10	90 sec
3. Barbell glute hip thrust		98	4-5	8-10	90 sec
4. Dumbbell walking lunge		60	3	20 total steps (10 on each leg)	60-90 sec
5. Forward sled drag (heavy load)		91	6-10	60 yd (55 m)	60-90 sec

Program Notes

- This training split can be run for 3 to 4 weeks.
- Increase training volume as your movement quality improves.
- Emphasize ingraining good motor patterns versus volume or load.
- This session should be separated from your other lower body sessions by 72 hours.

Exercise	Page	Sets	Reps	Rest
1. Barbell front box squat	81	5-8	1-5RM	2.5 min
2. Glute-ham raise	112	3-4	6-8	90 sec
3. Landmine lateral squat	72	3-4	6-8 each side	90 sec
4. Cable pull-through	94	3-4	15-20	60 sec
5. Backward sled drag (heavy load)	51	6	30 yd (27 m)	60-90 sec

BLOCK 3

Program Notes

- This training split can be run for 3 to 4 weeks.
- For the sumo stance deadlift against a band for dynamic effort, perform speed sets at 50 percent, 55 percent, 60 percent, and 65 percent of 1RM for 4 weeks.
- Increase training volume as your movement quality improves.
- Emphasize ingraining good motor patterns versus volume or load.
- This session should be separated from your other lower body sessions by 72 hours.

Exercise		Page	Sets	Reps	Rest
1. Sumo stance deadlift against a band for dynamic effort		123	6	2 @ 50% of 1RM + band tension	60 sec
2. Rear-foot elevated split squat		63	3-4	6-10 each side	90 sec
3. Medicine ball loaded back raise		101	4	15-20	60 sec
4. Backward sled drag (heavy load)		51	6	30 yd (27 m)	60-90 sec
5. Barbell tibia raise + calf raise		135	4	8-10	60 sec

Program Notes

- This training split can be run for 3 to 4 weeks.
- For the barbell front box squat, perform speed sets at 50 percent, 55 percent, 60 percent, and 65 percent of 1RM for 4 weeks.
- Increase training volume as your movement quality improves.
- Emphasize ingraining good motor patterns versus volume or load.
- This session should be separated from your other lower body sessions by 72 hours.

Exercise		Page	Sets	Reps	Rest
1. Barbell front box squat		81	5-8	1-5RM	2.5 min
2. Sumo stance Romanian deadlift with bands pulling forward		106	4-5	8-10	90 sec to 2 min
3. Landmine goblet reverse lunge		58	3-4	8-10 each side	60 sec
4. Single-leg glute hip thrust		96	2-3	12-15 each side	60 sec
5. Forward sled drag (heavy load)		91	6-10	60 yd (55 m)	60-90 sec

In conclusion, strength development requires a multifaceted approach in which all strengths are developed strategically in a concurrent training plan. In this case, the objective is to work both ends of the force-velocity curve: both the force component (submaximal effort training) and the velocity component (DE training) within the same cycle of training. Although there are varying opinions on whether it is prudent to train multiple aspects of strength within the same microcycles, from my professional experience it is not only possible but optimal for a large percentage of the population. To be clear, I am taking into consideration that the majority of people reading this book are likely very experienced in training bilateral movements and likely have at least five years of serious training under their belt. These approaches are certainly not for the beginner, who should aim first to achieve a high level of competency with foundational movement patterns and focus on one aspect of strength at a time.

Chapter 11

Athletic Performance Programs

The athletic training programs you'll find in this chapter are different in many ways from the other training plans in the book, although there are parallels to the hypertrophy and strength programs presented in the previous two chapters. A training program with an athletic performance focus needs to resemble the demands of your chosen sport with regard to the following:

- Energy systems development (ESD)
- Volume, selection, and intensity of plyometric exercises
- Your choice of strength methods

Does that mean that athletic training programs can't be used for general fitness? No, it does not; many former athletes enjoy keeping their competitive edge and like to train as if they were still competing as an athlete. If that's the case for you, keep in mind that your training methods should always align with your goals. For example, maximal effort (ME) training is something I use sparingly for myself and my clients who are former athletes because we still like to hit the occasional personal record on lifts. While ME training is a viable method for the right individual, going past the point of mechanical breakdown will increase the risk in the risk versus reward ratio, so it's not something that I use with most clients. Use the training methods that are appropriate for your goals and your sport.

MEETING THE DEMANDS OF YOUR SPORT

It's no mystery that athletic programs have the goal of improving performance and tailoring the programming to align with the demands of a sport or event make sense. However, coaches often make the mistake of going down the sport-specific rabbit hole trying to, in essence, reinvent the wheel. It is of my professional opinion that this is not the best way to train an athlete for their sport. Instead, it is prudent to rely on sound principles of programming such as foundational movement pattern development, strength development (maximal strength, explosive strength, and strength endurance), and aerobic fitness to improve recovery between sets and overall recoverability. The major difference in the programs found in this chapter versus other chapters in part III is the utilization of different methods to improve athletic performance. In this section, we will discuss those methods building upon what's already been discussed, such as maximal strength development, hypertrophy, and general physical preparedness (GPP).

Energy Systems Development

ESD is a critical aspect of any athletic performance program, along with understanding how to prioritize methods to improve the aerobic system and the anaerobic system applicable to the specificity of the sport. While this book is not meant to inform you on all of the methods that can be used to develop both the aerobic and anaerobic systems, it's important to know that the lower body strength programs provided in this book are a bridge to conditioning methods, meaning that they should align with the conditioning methods a coach chooses. For example, if athletes were performing an intensive ME lower body session on Monday followed by methods to improve the capacity of their glycolytic system on Tuesday, they may be at risk of overtraining due to the large neural demand created by these methods performed on back-to-back days. A better option would be to understand the neural load from each training session and use your conditioning sessions to bridge the gap between the main strength training sessions. Table 11.1 provides a sample ESD training template that would ensure optimal central nervous system recovery between sessions while still allowing athletes to improve their conditioning concurrently.

There is a time and a place for conditioning within these training programs, but methods cannot be haphazardly thrown in, and there should be a structure in place (as in table 11.1) to ensure optimal recovery between sessions.

Table 11.1 Sample ESD Training Template

Monday	Tuesday	Wednesday	Thursday	Friday	Saturday	Sunday
Maximal effort (lower)	Strongman-style endurance (aerobic)	Repeated effort (upper)	Cardiac output method (aerobic)	Dynamic effort (lower)	Dynamic effort (upper)	OFF

Plyometrics

Plyometric exercises are an important aspect of athletic programming because the application to the field of play is noteworthy. For instance, learning how to move explosively (explosive strength) and absorb force is not only necessary for all sports but an important factor for performance in sports. It's well established that the adaptations that take place in skeletal muscle from performing plyometrics are noticeable, but most strength professionals have questions around when plyometric exercises are included in strength programming, what variations to choose, and what are the proper volume prescriptions and rest intervals—all of which are covered in this book. (Please review chapter 8 for the physiology of plyometric training.)

Table 11.2 provides suggested volume prescriptions based upon your level of progress for the plyometric exercises you'll find in this chapter.

While these volume prescriptions are appropriate for most, you will also need to take into account your training age, training history, and muscle fiber dominance. (For example, an American football running back will present differently than an endurance athlete.)

It's also important to remember that more is not always better and that it always makes the most sense to start at the lower end of the volume prescription. The training programs in this chapter offer exercise

Table 11.2 Suggested Plyometric Exercise Volume Prescriptions for Athletic Performance Programs

	Sets	Reps	Rest	Total volume
Beginner	4	3	60 sec	12
Intermediate	8	3	45 sec	24
Advanced	10	3	30-45 sec	30

variations that increase in difficulty and training volume as you progress from beginner-intermediate to advanced with regard to age and training history.

Strength Training Methods

As discussed in chapter 3, there are a number of viable methods of optimal strength development. (Please review chapter 3 for the complete breakdown.) The programming in this book uses the following:

- *ME method:* one repetition for maximal load
- *Repeated effort method:* hypertrophy-style work performed in the 8- to 15-rep range with single-joint movement patterns
- *Submaximal effort method:* multiple-repetition maxes with bilateral lifts or heavy sets building in weight across multiple sets (i.e., build to a heavy five in five sets)
- *Dynamic effort method and explosive strength:* submaximal loading with the intent of movement velocity
- *GPP work:* performed using a variety of sled drag variations and loaded carries

All of the methods used in this book serve as the foundation to develop maximal strength, explosive strength, efficient foundational movement patterns (e.g., squat, single-leg, hip hinge), and GPP to ensure the athlete is well-rounded and resilient.

ATHLETIC PERFORMANCE PROGRAMS

While this book focuses on strategies for the lower body, knowing where to place these training days within the training cycle is important so that you're including upper body–centric days as well as ESD. Table 11.3 shows five training split options that will allow for proper nervous system recovery between sessions. These splits assume that you use a concurrent approach to training (i.e., training multiple qualities of both strength and conditioning within the same week of training).

This chapter includes four blocks of beginner-intermediate programming and four blocks of advanced programming. Despite this separation into beginner-intermediate and advanced programs, the connection between all three levels of programming is stronger than you might think because the primary goal across all levels is to train foundational movement patterns. The difference between beginner, intermediate, and advanced lies in the complexity of exercise variations, the choice in training methods (i.e., maximal effort versus submaximal effort), and the level of volume prescribed.

Table 11.3 Sample Training Split Options for Athletic Performance Training

	Day 1	Day 2	Day 3	Day 4	Day 5	Day 6	Day 7
Training split option 1	Lower	ESD	Upper	ESD	Lower	Upper	OFF
Training split option 2	Upper	Lower	ESD	Upper	Lower	ESD	OFF
Training split option 3	Upper	ESD	Lower	ESD	Upper	ESD	Lower
Training split option 4	Lower	ESD	Upper	ESD	Total	OFF	OFF
Training split option 5	Total	ESD	Total	ESD	Total	ESD	OFF

BEGINNER-INTERMEDIATE PROGRAM
WITH ATHLETIC PERFORMANCE EMPHASIS

BLOCK 1

Program Notes
- This training split can be run for 3 to 4 weeks.
- For the trap bar deadlift, build to a heavy 3 to 5 reps in 5 sets.
- Increase training volume as your movement quality improves.
- Emphasize ingraining good motor patterns versus volume or load.
- This session should be separated from your other lower body sessions by 72 hours.

Exercise	Page	Sets	Reps	Rest
1. Seated dynamic box jump	166	5	3	45-60 sec
2. Trap bar deadlift	116	5	Build to a heavy 5 or 5RM	2-3 min
3. Goblet box squat	75	3-4	10-12	60 sec
4. Single-leg glute hip thrust	96	2-3	12-15 each side	60 sec
5. 1-1/4 dumbbell split squat	54	2-3	12-15 each side (1 full ROM rep + 1/4 rep at the bottom of each rep = 1 rep)	45-60 sec

Program Notes

- This training split can be run for 3 to 4 weeks.
- For the barbell front box squat, perform 8 sets × 3 reps for speed (dynamic effort using 50 to 60 percent of 1RM back squat to 16-inch [40 cm] box). Each week, add 3 to 5 percent to your load while still maintaining bar velocity.
- Increase training volume as your movement quality improves.
- Emphasize ingraining good motor patterns versus volume or load.
- This session should be separated from your other lower body sessions by 72 hours.

Exercise		Page	Sets	Reps	Rest
1. Kettlebell squat jump		170	4	4	45-60 sec
2. Barbell front box squat		81	5-8	1-5RM	2.5 min
3. Glute-ham raise		112	3-4	6-8	90 sec
4. Goblet squat		76	3-4	12-15	60 sec
5. Cable pull-through		94	3-4	15-20	60 sec

BLOCK 3

Program Notes

- This training split can be run for 3 to 4 weeks.
- For the Anderson front squat, build to a heavy 3 set with pins so you start at parallel. Each week, build to a heavy 4 in week 1; a heavy 3 in week 2; a heavy 2 in week 3; and a heavy 1 in week 4. If possible, use accommodating resistance (AR) for your Anderson front squat rep max on weeks 3 and 4.
- Increase training volume as your movement quality improves.
- Emphasize ingraining good motor patterns versus volume or load.
- This session should be separated from your other lower body sessions by 72 hours.

Exercise	Page	Sets	Reps	Rest
1. Seated dynamic vertical jump	164	5	3	45-60 sec
2. Anderson front squat	78	Build in weight over the course of 5 sets	5RM	2.5 min
3. Band-assisted glute-ham raise	114	4	5-7	90 sec
4. Dumbbell walking lunge	60	3	20 total steps (10 on each leg)	60-90 sec
5. Lateral sled drag (moderate load)	129	6	30 yd (27 m) each side	60-90 sec

Program Notes

- This training split can be run for 3 to 4 weeks.
- For the barbell front box squat, use a 16-inch (40 cm) box and use 60 percent, 63 percent, 66 percent, and 70 percent of 1RM back squat; if possible, use AR and drop the percentages to 45 percent, 50 percent, 55 percent, and 60 percent.
- Increase training volume as your movement quality improves.
- Emphasize ingraining good motor patterns versus volume or load.
- This session should be separated from your other lower body sessions by 72 hours.

Exercise	Page	Sets	Reps	Rest
1. Barbell squat jump	174	5	4 @ 20%-30% of back squat 1RM	60 sec
2. Barbell front box squat	81	5-8	1-5RM	2.5 min
3. Barbell glute hip thrust	98	4-5	8-10	90 sec
4. Landmine lateral squat	72	3-4	6-8 each side	90 sec
5. Forward sled drag (heavy load)	91	6-10	60 yd (55 m)	60-90 sec

ADVANCED PROGRAM WITH ATHLETIC PERFORMANCE EMPHASIS

BLOCK 1

Program Notes

- This training split can be run for 3 to 4 weeks.
- For the trap bar deadlift, build to a heavy 4 in week 1, a heavy 3 in week 2, a heavy 2 in week 3, and a 1RM in week 4.
- Increase training volume as your movement quality improves.
- Emphasize ingraining good motor patterns versus volume or load.
- This session should be separated from your other lower body sessions by 72 hours.

Exercise	Page	Sets	Reps	Rest
1. Kneeling jump	187	6	3	60 sec
2. Trap bar deadlift	116	5	Build to a rep max	2-3 min
3. Landmine lateral squat	72	3-4	6-8 each side	90 sec
4. Forward sled drag (heavy load)	91	6-10	60 yd (55 m)	60-90 sec
5. Banded pull-through	154	4	25	45-60 sec

Program Notes

- This training split can be run for 3 to 4 weeks.
- For the barbell front box squat, build to 4RM in week 1, 3RM in week 2, heavy 2RM in week 3, and 1RM in week 4. If possible, use AR for your rep max on weeks 3 and 4.
- Increase training volume as your movement quality improves.
- Emphasize ingraining good motor patterns versus volume or load.
- This session should be separated from your other lower body sessions by 72 hours.

Exercise	Page	Sets	Reps	Rest
1. Dumbbell squat jump + box jump	180	5	2 (1 dumbbell squat jump + 1 box jump)	60 sec
2. Barbell front box squat	81	5-8	Build to a 1RM	2.5 min
3. Loaded glute-ham raise	115	4	6-8	90 sec
4. Landmine lateral squat	72	3-4	6-8 each side	90 sec
5. Backward sled drag (heavy load)	51	6	30 yd (27 m)	60-90 sec

BLOCK 3

Program Notes

- This training split can be run for 3 to 4 weeks.
- For the sumo stance deadlift against a band for dynamic effort, perform speed sets at 50 percent, 55 percent, 60 percent, and 65 percent of 1RM for 4 weeks.
- Increase training volume as your movement quality improves.
- Emphasize ingraining good motor patterns versus volume or load.
- This session should be separated from your other lower body sessions by 72 hours.

Exercise	Page	Sets	Reps	Rest
1. Single-leg box jump	176	6	2 each side	45-60 sec
2. Sumo stance deadlift against a band for dynamic effort	123	6	2 @ 50% of 1RM + band tension	60 sec
3. Rear-foot elevated split squat	63	3-4	6-10 each side	90 sec
4. 45-degree back raise	100	3-4	12-15	60 sec
5. Backward sled drag (heavy load)	51	6	30 yd (27 m)	60-90 sec

Program Notes

- This training split can be run for 3 to 4 weeks.
- For the sumo stance deadlift against a band for dynamic effort, perform speed sets at 50 percent, 55 percent, 60 percent, and 65 percent of 1RM for 4 weeks.
- For the barbell front box squat clusters, build to a heavy 6 (a load that is heavy for 6 reps but not necessarily a 6RM) and rest for 2 minutes between sets. Then perform 3 cluster sets of 3 reps, rerack, and rest for 20 seconds. Next, do 2 reps, rerack, and rest for 20 seconds. Finally, do 1 rep, rerack, and rest for 3 minutes. This should be done at 80 to 85 percent of 1RM front squat.
- Increase training volume as your movement quality improves.
- Emphasize ingraining good motor patterns versus volume or load.
- This session should be separated from your other lower body sessions by 72 hours.

Exercise	Page	Sets	Reps	Rest
1. Single-leg box jump	176	6	2 each side	45-60 sec
2. Sumo stance deadlift against a band for dynamic effort	123	6	2 @ 50% of 1RM + band tension	60 sec
3. Barbell front box squat clusters	83	3	3.2.1 (20 sec)	3 min
4. Forward sled drag (heavy load)	91	6-10	60 yd (55 m)	60-90 sec
5. Seated single-leg banded hamstring curl	138	5	25 each side	As needed

In conclusion, athletic performance training programs carry many of the tenets of other programs discussed in this book. Programs with different goals must still rely on basic principles. For example, effective hypertrophy training will improve muscular imbalance and add lean tissue to your frame. You must allow for proper nervous system recovery in between sessions in order to prevent overtraining. We provide training templates that allow for the greatest number of days between the most demanding training sessions so that your body can fully recover. Adding reliable and effective explosive strength work via plyometrics and repeated effort work via single-joint exercises—with adjustments to volume prescriptions, frequency, and exercise selection—will help you reach your athletic performance goals.

Chapter 12

At-Home Training Programs

Training from home has gained popularity, especially since 2020, when people were unable to access commercial gyms because of the worldwide pandemic. Having the freedom to train when you want and how you want, paired with the convenience of being in your own home, is attractive to many and something that I have personally taken advantage of for the last five years. If you are already familiar with how to perform big compound movements, you may be self-sufficient and able to train on your own. You can feel empowered and confident in being able to challenge yourself without the need for a coach or the pressure of competing against your peers.

The training programs in this chapter are designed to be time-efficient and use a limited amount of equipment—a barbell, resistance bands, a landmine, kettlebells, and dumbbells. You should have weights available that support your current strength levels. If you do need to add to your equipment, you can do so with a relatively small investment and make these programs work quite well for you from the comfort of your own home. And if you're new to training from home, you may never go back to training at a commercial gym; at-home training is really convenient!

BUILDING A HOME GYM

Home gyms have become quite popular due to the freedom and convenience they provide. Moreover, former athletes are perfect candidates for training on their own—most are familiar with how to perform big compound movements and over the years have become self-sufficient in terms of training. The questions that typically arise when building a home gym center around what equipment one needs and why, so I've compiled two lists: the "must-haves" and the "nice-to-haves." Keep in mind that you do not have to spend an exorbitant amount of money to sufficiently train from home—quite the contrary—and considering the cost of a gym membership, travel time to and from a gym, and associated fuel costs, what you'll save may make up for the initial investment. Of course, nothing here is mandatory, and you can certainly get away with a lot less. (Many of the programs in this chapter require less than what's recommended here.)

Must-Haves

- *Squat rack.* A rack can serve a number of purposes vital to your training. For instance, you'll want a rack that allows you to pull rack deadlifts, perform multiple-grip pull-ups, perform a variety of exercises off of pins (Anderson squats, pin presses, etc.), and set up bands for accommodating resistance (AR).
- *Barbell.* This one goes without saying, but do yourself a favor and invest in a good barbell because you'll have it for the rest of your life.
- *Dumbbells.* The value of having multiple sizes of dumbbells on hand is clear, but a few sets can go a long way in keeping your training interesting and your progression consistent.
- *Kettlebells.* This is another piece of equipment where a few will likely be all you need to keep your training interesting.
- *Bands.* Having a few sets of bands with different thicknesses will allow you to train even when you're away from home and also adds the ability to use AR, which has a number of great benefits already covered in chapter 3.
- *Pulling sled.* The sled is one of the most versatile tools known to man for strength, conditioning, and recovery measures. For less than 100 dollars, you'll have a training tool that will take your training to the next level. (The sled is utilized in most of the programs in this book for good reason.)

- *Landmine.* Another incredibly versatile tool that can cover just about all of your training needs, including lunge variations, complexes, squats, presses, and more.
- *Bench.* Having an adjustable bench is definitely an added luxury— you can create a slight decline or incline by simply elevating the front or back of the bench on a few bumper plates, adding variability to pressing exercises. Moreover, the bench is about 16 inches (40 cm) high, which is a nice height to perform box squats with as well.
- *Plyometric box.* This is another piece of equipment that may not seem absolutely necessary, but if you're planning on effectively training your fast-twitch muscle fibers, a plyometric box is definitely a must-have.
- *Storage.* With all your new equipment, you'll likely need to invest in some type of storage for the smaller equipment. Most areas that people allot for their home gyms are small, so every bit of area counts.

Nice-to-Haves

- *Safety squat bar.* This one is higher up on the list than you may think mainly because this bar has been a game changer in terms of pain-free squatting—the camber of the bar, the ability to use the handles, and the variety of different exercises outside of just squatting you can perform with it (like pressing) provide a massive return on investment.
- *Chains.* These are definitely not a necessity but can add variety to your routine, improve multiple levels of strength, and prevent injury compared to only using straight barbell weight.
- *Fatbells.* The fatbell is a variation of the dumbbell where the weight is more symmetrical. These can turn normal exercises like presses into new variations.
- *Pushing sled.* This is an incredible conditioning tool that much like the pulling sled can serve both strength and conditioning purposes when used strategically.
- *Air bike.* You'll likely want to have at least one piece of conditioning equipment like an air bike at some point. This will give you the ability to perform conditioning work inside when the weather does not permit outside work.

In short, building your home gym certainly doesn't have to break the bank out of the gate—stick with the first five things on the must-have list to get you started, and slowly build from there. The best part is that you can build over time while you discern your individual needs.

AT-HOME TRAINING PROGRAMS

While this book focuses on strategies for the lower body, knowing where to place these training days within the training cycle is important so that you're including upper body–centric days as well as energy systems development (ESD). For most people that are training at home, ESD can be as simple as going for a light jog or walk, depending on your current level of ability. Table 12.1 shows five training split options that will allow for proper nervous system recovery between sessions. These splits also assume that you use a concurrent approach to training (i.e., training multiple qualities of both strength and conditioning within the same week of training).

This chapter includes four blocks of beginner-intermediate programming and four blocks of advanced programming. Despite this separation into beginner-intermediate and advanced programs, the connection between all three levels of programming is stronger than you might think because the primary goal across all levels is to train foundational movement patterns. The difference between beginner, intermediate, and advanced lies in the complexity of exercise variations, the choice in training methods (i.e., maximal effort versus submaximal effort), and the level of volume prescribed.

Table 12.1 Sample Training Split Options for At-Home Training

	Day 1	Day 2	Day 3	Day 4	Day 5	Day 6	Day 7
Training split option 1	Lower	ESD	Upper	ESD	Lower	Upper	OFF
Training split option 2	Upper	Lower	ESD	Upper	Lower	ESD	OFF
Training split option 3	Upper	ESD	Lower	ESD	Upper	ESD	Lower
Training split option 4	Lower	ESD	Upper	ESD	Total	OFF	OFF
Training split option 5	Total	ESD	Total	ESD	Total	ESD	OFF

BEGINNER-INTERMEDIATE PROGRAM WITH AT-HOME TRAINING EMPHASIS

BLOCK 1

Program Notes

Exercises are done as supersets where you perform the *a* exercise, rest 45 seconds, and then perform the *b* exercise, going back and forth to complete all sets of that pairing before moving to the next numbered pair of exercises.

Exercise		Page	Sets	Reps	Rest
1a. Barbell front box squat		81	4	1-5RM	2.5 min
1b. Banded pull-through		154	4	25	45-60 sec
2a. Single-leg landmine Romanian deadlift		103	2-3	8-10 each side	60 sec
2b. Goblet lateral squat		73	2-3	8-10 each side	90 sec
3a. Single-leg hinged-back banded abduction		148	3	5 each side	60 sec
3b. Single-leg dumbbell calf raise		131	3	8-10 each side	60 sec

Program Notes

Exercises are done as supersets where you perform the *a* exercise, rest 45 seconds, and then perform the *b* exercise, going back and forth to complete all sets of that pairing before moving to the next numbered pair of exercises.

Exercise		Page	Sets	Reps	Rest
1a. Sumo stance Romanian deadlift with bands pulling forward		106	3-4	8-10	90 sec to 2 min
1b. Goblet squat		76	3-4	12-15	60 sec
2a. Barbell glute hip thrust		98	3-4	8-10	90 sec
2b. Single-leg dumbbell calf raise		131	3-4	8-10 each side	60 sec
3a. Banded pull-through		154	3-4	25	45-60 sec
3b. Dumbbell split squat		53	3-4	8-10 each side	60 sec

BEGINNER-INTERMEDIATE PROGRAM
WITH AT-HOME TRAINING EMPHASIS *(continued)*

BLOCK 3

Program Notes

Exercises are done as supersets where you perform the *a* exercise, rest 45 seconds, and then perform the *b* exercise, going back and forth to complete all sets of that pairing before moving to the next numbered pair of exercises.

Exercise	Page	Sets	Reps	Rest
1a. Trap bar Romanian deadlift	117	3-4	8-10	90 sec to 2 min
1b. Landmine lateral squat	72	3-4	6-8 each side	90 sec
2a. Band-resisted glute bridge	142	3-4	8-10	60 sec
2b. Rear-foot elevated split squat	63	3-4	6-10 each side	90 sec
3a. Banded pull-through	154	3-4	25	45-60 sec
3b. Single-leg dumbbell calf raise	131	3-4	8-10 each side	60 sec

Program Notes

- This block of programming does *not* include any supersets.
- Perform 2 to 3 warm-up sets and then the listed number of work sets.
- For the barbell front box squat, build to a moderate load using a 16-inch (40 cm) box.

Exercise		Page	Sets	Reps	Rest
1. Barbell front box squat		81	5-8	1-5RM	2.5 min
2. Barbell glute hip thrust		98	4-5	8-10	90 sec
3. Landmine lateral squat		72	3-4	6-8 each side	90 sec
4. Seated double-leg banded hamstring curl		140	4	20-30	60 sec
5. Single-leg dumbbell calf raise		131	3-4	8-10 each side	60 sec

ADVANCED PROGRAM WITH AT-HOME TRAINING EMPHASIS

BLOCK 1

Program Notes

Exercises are done as supersets where you perform the *a* exercise, rest 45 seconds, and then perform the *b* exercise, going back and forth to complete all sets of that pairing before moving to the next numbered pair of exercises.

Exercise	Page	Sets	Reps	Rest
1a. 1-1/4 front squat	84	4	4RM (1 full ROM rep + 1/4 rep at the bottom of each rep = 1 rep)	2.5 min
1b. Banded pull-through	154	4	25	45-60 sec
2a. Barbell glute hip thrust	98	3-4	8-10	90 sec
2b. Landmine goblet reverse lunge	58	3-4	8-10 each side	60 sec
3a. Barbell tibia raise + calf raise	135	3	8-10	60 sec
3b. X-band walk + banded good morning	156	3	5 left walks + 5 right walks + 5 good mornings	60 sec

Program Notes

Exercises are done as supersets where you perform the *a* exercise, rest 45 seconds, and then perform the *b* exercise, going back and forth to complete all sets of that pairing before moving to the next numbered pair of exercises.

Exercise	Page	Sets	Reps	Rest
1a. Sumo stance Romanian deadlift with bands pulling forward	106	3-4	8-10	90 sec to 2 min
1b. Goblet squat	76	3-4	12-15	60 sec
2a. Barbell glute hip thrust	98	3-4	8-10	90 sec
2b. Single-leg dumbbell calf raise	131	3-4	8-10 each side	60 sec
3a. Banded pull-through	154	3	25	45-60 sec
3b. Single-leg hinged-back banded abduction with support	149	3	5 each side	60 sec

BLOCK 3

Program Notes

Exercises are done as supersets where you perform the *a* exercise, rest 45 seconds, and then perform the *b* exercise, going back and forth to complete all sets of that pairing before moving to the next numbered pair of exercises.

Exercise	Page	Sets	Reps	Rest
1a. Single-leg landmine Romanian deadlift	103	3-4	8-10 each side	60 sec
1b. 1-1/4 front squat	84	3-4	4RM (1 full ROM rep + 1/4 rep at the bottom of each rep = 1 rep)	2.5 min
2a. Band-resisted glute bridge	142	3	8-10	60 sec
2b. Landmine reverse lunge	57	3	8-10 each side	60 sec
3a. Banded pull-through	154	4	25	45-60 sec
3b. Single-leg dumbbell calf raise	131	4	8-10 each side	60 sec

Program Notes

- This block of programming does *not* include any supersets.
- Perform 2 to 3 warm-up sets and then the listed number of work sets.
- For the Anderson front squat, build to a 5RM (or a heavy 5) in 5 sets.

Exercise	Page	Sets	Reps	Rest
1. Anderson front squat	78	Build in weight over the course of 5 sets	5RM	2.5 min
2. 1-1/2 single-leg glute hip thrust	97	3-4	8-10 each side (1 full ROM rep + 1/2 rep at the bottom of each rep = 1 rep)	60 sec
3. Landmine goblet reverse lunge	58	3-4	8-10 each side	60 sec
4. Seated single-leg banded hamstring curl	138	5	25 each side	As needed
5. Barbell tibia raise + calf raise	135	4	8-10	60 sec

In conclusion, training from home certainly does not have to be boring and can be as effective as going to a commercial gym. Those who are willing to invest in a home gym are a special breed—there is no doubt that you take your health and training seriously. The training programs in this chapter are options I've provided to actual clients who train from home. If you want to train at home long-term, many of the other training programs listed in chapters 9, 10, and 11 will become great options for you as you build your collection of home gym equipment.

REFERENCES

Contreras, Bret. 2019. *Glute Lab*. Victory Belt.

Cooper, Nicholas A., Kelsey M. Scavo, Kyle J. Strickland, Natti Tipayamongkol, Jeffrey D. Nicholson, Dennis C. Bewyer, Kathleen A. Sluka, et al. 2016. "Prevalence of Gluteus Medius Weakness in People With Chronic Low Back Pain Compared to Healthy Controls." *European Spine Journal* 25 (4): 1258-65. https://pubmed.ncbi.nlm.nih.gov/26006705.

Cormie, Prue, Michael R. McGuigan, and Robert U. Newton. 2011. "Developing Maximal Neuromuscular Power: Part 2—Training Considerations for Improving Maximal Power Production." *Sports Medicine* 41: 125-46.

French, Duncan. 2016. "Adaptations to Anaerobic Training Programs." In *Essentials of Strength Training and Conditioning*, edited by G. Gregory Haff and N. Travis Triplett, 87-112. Champaign, IL: Human Kinetics.

Haff, G. Gregory. 2016. "Periodization." In *Essentials of Strength Training and Conditioning*, edited by G. Gregory Haff and N. Travis Triplett, 583-604. Champaign, IL: Human Kinetics.

Haff, G. Gregory, and Tudor Bompa. 2009. *Periodization*. 5th ed. Champaign, IL: Human Kinetics.

International Sports Sciences Association. n.d. "Setting Fitness Goals is Essential to Long-Term Success." www.issaonline.com/blog/index.cfm/2019/setting-fitness-goals-is-essential--to-long-term-success.

Kraemer, William J., Jakob L. Vingren, and Barry A. Spiering. 2016. "Endocrine Responses to Resistance Exercise." In *Essentials of Strength Training and Conditioning*, edited by G. Gregory Haff and N. Travis Triplett, 65-86. Champaign, IL: Human Kinetics.

McGill, Stuart. 2015. *Back Mechanic*. Backfit Pro.

Netter, Frank H. 2018. *Atlas of Human Anatomy*. 7th ed. Philadelphia, PA: Elsevier Saunders.

Potach, David, and Donald A. Chu. 2016. "Program Design and Technique for Plyometric Training." In *Essentials of Strength Training and Conditioning*, edited by G. Gregory Haff and N. Travis Triplett, 471-520. Champaign, IL: Human Kinetics.

Rohen, Johannes W., Chihiro Yokochi, and Elke Lütjen-Drecoll. 2012. *Color Atlas of Anatomy*. 7th ed. Philadelphia, PA: Wolters Kluwer.

Schoenfeld, Brad J. 2021. *Science and Development Muscle Hypertrophy*. Champaign, IL: Human Kinetics.

Simmons, Louie. 2015. *Special Strength Development For All Sports*. Action Printing.

Tortora, Gerard J., and Bryan H. Derrickson. 2016. *Principles of Anatomy and Physiology*. 15th ed. Hoboken, NJ: Wiley.

Verkhoshansky, Yuri, and Mel Siff. 2009. *Supertraining*. 6th ed. Rome: Verkhoshansky.

Zatsiorsky, Vladimir M., William J. Kraemer, and Andrew C. Fry. 2021. *Science and Practice of Strength Training*. 3rd ed. Champaign, IL: Human Kinetics.

ABOUT THE AUTHOR

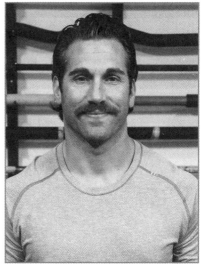

Jason Brown has a master of science degree in exercise physiology and holds the Certified Strength and Conditioning Specialist (CSCS) credential. He is a Conjugate Method expert and is one of the few professionals certified as a Special Strength Coach under the legendary Louie Simmons of Westside Barbell. After owning his own CrossFit facility for six years, he started Jason Brown Coaching, an online programming business that provides programming to CrossFit affiliates and strength and conditioning facilities around the world. He holds CrossFit certifications in powerlifting, mobility, gymnastics, coaches' prep, CrossFit Level 2, endurance, and Olympic lifting.

With more than 17 years of experience in the fitness industry, Brown specializes in providing programming to both individuals and facilities as well as education to strength and conditioning professionals. He presents for the National Strength and Conditioning Association (NSCA) and has published hundreds of articles with platforms such as EliteFTS, T Nation, DrJohnRusin.com, and ThibArmy (Christian Thibaudeau). Brown is also a combat veteran of Operation Enduring Freedom and a father of three.

You read the book—now complete the companion CE exam to earn continuing education credit!

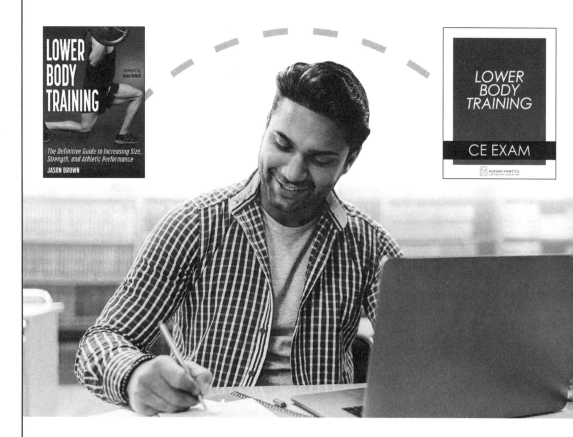

Find and purchase the companion CE exam here:
US.HumanKinetics.com/collections/CE-Exam
Canada.HumanKinetics.com/collections/CE-Exam

50% off the companion CE exam with this code

LBT2023

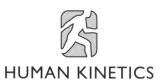

HUMAN KINETICS